FOOD SECURITY AND CHILD MALNUTRITION

The Impact on Health, Growth, and Well-Being

FOOD SECURITY AND CHILD MALNUTRITION

The Impact on Health, Growth, and Well-Being

Edited by
Areej Hassan, MD, MPH

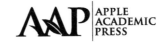

Apple Academic Press Inc. | Apple Academic Press Inc.
3333 Mistwell Crescent | 9 Spinnaker Way
Oakville, ON L6L 0A2 | Waretown, NJ 08758
Canada | USA

©2017 by Apple Academic Press, Inc.

First issued in paperback 2021

Exclusive worldwide distribution by CRC Press, a member of Taylor & Francis Group
No claim to original U.S. Government works

ISBN 13: 978-1-77-463687-9 (pbk)
ISBN 13: 978-1-77-188493-8 (hbk)

Library and Archives Canada Cataloguing in Publication

Food security and child malnutrition : the impact on health, growth, and well-being / edited by Areej Hassan, MD, MPH.

Includes bibliographical references and index.
Issued in print and electronic formats.
ISBN 978-1-77188-493-8 (hardcover).--ISBN 978-1-77188-494-5 (pdf)
1. Children--Nutrition. 2. Food security. I. Hassan, Areej, editor

RJ206.F63 2016   613.2083   C2016-906549-9   C2016-906550-2

Library of Congress Cataloging-in-Publication Data

Names: Hassan, Areej, editor.
Title: Food security and child malnutrition : the impact on health, growth, and well-being / editor, Areej Hassan.
Description: Toronto ; New Jersey : Apple Academic Press, 2017. | Includes bibliographical references and index.
Identifiers: LCCN 2016050043 (print) | LCCN 2016051015 (ebook) | ISBN 9781771884938 (hardcover : alk. paper) | ISBN 9781315365749 (ebook)
Subjects: | MESH: Child Nutrition Disorders | Food Supply | Health Status Classification:
LCC RJ206 (print) | LCC RJ206 (ebook) | NLM WS 130 | DDC 362.1963/9--dc23
LC record available at https://lccn.loc.gov/2016050043

Apple Academic Press also publishes its books in a variety of electronic formats. Some content that appears in print may not be available in electronic format. For information about Apple Academic Press products, visit our website at **www.appleacademicpress.com** and the CRC Press website at **www.crc-press.com**

About the Editor

Areej Hassan, MD, MPH

Areej Hassan, MD, MPH, is an attending in the Division of Adolescent/Young Adult Medicine at Boston Children's Hospital and Assistant Professor of Pediatrics at Harvard Medical School, Boston, Massachusetts. She completed her residency training in Pediatrics at Brown University before her fellowship at BCH. In addition to primary care, Dr. Hassan focuses her clinical interests on reproductive endocrinology and global health. She also maintains an active role in medical education and has particular interest in building and developing innovative teaching tools through open educational resources. She currently teaches, consults, and is involved in pediatric and adolescent curricula development at multiple sites abroad in Central America and Southeast Asia.

Contents

List of Contributors

Shamsir Ahmed
International Centers for Diarrheal Disease Research

Tahmeed Ahmed
International Centers for Diarrheal Disease Research

Kathleen W. Barrett
Arkansas Children's Hospital

Tefera Belachew
Department of Population and Family Health, Nutrition Unit, College of Public Health and Medical Sciences, Jimma University; Department of Food Safety and Food Quality, Faculty of Bioscience Engineering, Ghent University.

Pascal Bessong
University of Venda

Jasmin Bhawra
School of Public Health and Health Systems, University of Waterloo

Zulfiqar A. Bhutta
Division of Women and Child Health, Aga Khan University

Michel Boivin
Université Laval, Québec, Canada

Amanda Breen
Drexel University School of Public Health

Daniel Burnier
Institute of Population Health, University of Ottawa

Laura Caulfield
Program in Global Disease Epidemiology and Control and Division of Human Nutrition, Bloomberg School of Public Health, Johns Hopkins University

Mwatasa Changoma
Nagasaki University Institute of Tropical Medicine (NUITM) - Kenya Medical Research Institute (KEMRI) Project

Jean-François Chastang
INSERM U1018, Centre for research in Epidemiology and Population Health, Epidemiology of occupational and social determinants of health, F-94807, Villejuif, France; Université de Versailles Saint-Quentin, UMRS 1018, France

William Checkley
Fogarty International Center, National Institutes of Health; Division of Pulmonary and Critical Care, School of Medicine, Johns Hopkins University; Program in Global Disease Epidemiology and Control and Division of Human Nutrition, Bloomberg School of Public Health, Johns Hopkins University

John T. Cook
Boston University School of Medicine

Martin J. Cooke
School of Public Health and Health Systems, University of Waterloo; Department of Sociology and Legal Studies, University of Waterloo

Sylvana M. Côté
INSERM U669, Maison de Solenn, Université Paris-Sud and Université Paris-Descartes, 97 Bd du Port Royal, F-75679 Paris, France; International Laboratory for Child and Adolescent Mental Health, Research Group on Children's Psychosocial Maladjustment, University of Montreal, Montreal, Canada

Stephanie Ettinger de Cuba
Boston University School of Public Health

Colleen Davison
Department of Public Health Sciences, Queen's UniversityKGH Clinical Research Centre, Kingston General Hospital

Lise Dubois
Faculty of Medicine, University of Ottawa, Institute of Population Health

Bruno Falissard
INSERM U669, Maison de Solenn, Université Paris-Sud and Université Paris-Descartes, 97 Bd du Port Royal, F-75679 Paris, France

Kristin Fox
Sir Arthur Lewis Institute of Social Sciences and Economic Studies, University of the West Indies

Damion Francis
Epidemiology Research Unit- TMRI, University of the West Indies

Deborah A. Frank
Boston University School of Medicine

Cédric Galéra
Service de Pédopsychiatrie universitaire, Hôpital Charles-Perrens, Université Victor Ségalen Bordeaux 2, Bordeaux, France

Abebe Gebremariam
Department of Population and Family Health, Nutrition Unit, College of Public Health and Medical Sciences, Jimma University

Manon Girard
Institute of Population Health, University of Ottawa

Shelley L. H. Gonneville
Métis Nation of Ontario

Georgiana Gordon-Strachan
Faculty of Medical Sciences, Deans Office, University of the West Indies

Craig Hadley
Department of Anthropology, Emory University

Rhona Hanning
School of Public Health and Health Systems, University of Waterloo

Sheryl L. Hendriks
Institute for Food, Nutrition and Well-being, University of Pretoria

Munirul Islam
International Centers for Diarrheal Disease Research

Sushil John
Christian Medical College

Katherine M. Joyce
Northeast Ohio Medical University

Caroline W. Kabiru
African Population and Health Research Center; University of the Witwatersrand, School of Public Health

Ngianga-bakwin Kandala
Department of Population Health, Luxembourg Institute of Health; Department of Mathematics and Information sciences, Faculty of Engineering and Environment, Northumbria University

Satoshi Kaneko
Graduate School of International Health Development, Nagasaki University; Department of Eco-epidemiology, Institute of Tropical Medicine, Nagasaki University

Mohamed Karama
Graduate School of International Health Development, Nagasaki University; Centre for Public Health Research, Kenya Medical Research Institute (KEMRI)

Wondwosen Kasahun
Department of Epidemiology and Biostatistics, College of Public Health and Medical Sciences, Jimma University

Patrick Kolsteren
Department of Food Safety and Food Quality, Faculty of Bioscience Engineering, Ghent University; Nutrition and Child Health Unit, Department of Public Health, Institute of Tropical Medicine

Margaret Kosek
Program in Global Disease Epidemiology and Control and Division of Human Nutrition, Bloomberg School of Public Health, Johns Hopkins University

Aldo Lima
Federal University of Ceara

David Lindstrom
Department of Sociology, Brown University

Masaki Matsumura
Graduate School of International Health Development, Nagasaki University; Liaison Center for International Education, Nagasaki University

Monica McGrath
Fogarty International Center, National Institutes of Health; Program in Global Disease Epidemiology and Control and Division of Human Nutrition, Bloomberg School of Public Health, Johns Hopkins University

Maria Melchior
INSERM U1018, Centre for research in Epidemiology and Population Health, Epidemiology of occupational and social determinants of health, F-94807, Villejuif, France; Université de Versailles Saint-Quentin, UMRS 1018, France

Valerie Michaelson
School of Religion, Queen's University

Mark Miller
Fogarty International Center, National Institutes of Health

Maurice Mutisya
African Population and Health Research Center; University of the Witwatersrand, School of Public Health

Cebisa Nesamvuni
University of Venda

Moses Waithanji Ngware
African Population and Health Research Center; University of the Witwatersrand, School of Public Health

Grace Paik
University of Maryland School of Medicine

William Pickett
Department of Public Health Sciences, Queen's University

Stephanie Psaki
Fogarty International Center, National Institutes of Health; Program in Global Disease Epidemiology and Control and Division of Human Nutrition, Bloomberg School of Public Health, Johns Hopkins University

Bianca Pullen
Boston Medical Center

Stephanie Richard
Fogarty International Center, National Institutes of Health; Program in Global Disease Epidemiology and Control and Division of Human Nutrition, Bloomberg School of Public Health, Johns Hopkins University

Natasha Rishi
Boston Medical Center

Ashley Schiffmiller
Boston Medical Center

Jessica Seidman
Fogarty International Center, National Institutes of Health; Program in Global Disease Epidemiology and Control and Division of Human Nutrition, Bloomberg School of Public Health, Johns Hopkins University

Chisa Shinsugi
Graduate School of International Health Development, Nagasaki University; Department of Human Ecology, Graduate School of Medicine, The University of Tokyo

Prakash Shrestha
Institute of Medicine

Erling Svensen
University of Bergen

Junichi Tanaka
Department of Eco-epidemiology, Institute of Tropical Medicine, Nagasaki University; Department of Nursing, Graduate School of Biomedical Sciences, Nagasaki University

Fabiola Tatone-Tokuda
Institute of Population Health, University of Ottawa

Richard E. Tremblay
INSERM U669, Maison de Solenn, Université Paris-Sud and Université Paris-Descartes, 97 Bd du Port Royal,
F-75679 Paris, France; International Laboratory for Child and Adolescent Mental Health, Research Group on
Children's Psychosocial Maladjustment, University of Montreal, Montreal, Canada

Piotr Wilk
Schulich School of Medicine and Dentistry, Western University

Rainford Wilks
Epidemiology Research Unit- TMRI, University of the West Indies

Acknowledgments and How to Cite

The editor and publisher thank each of the authors who contributed to this book. Many of the chapters in this book were previously published elsewhere. To cite the work contained in this book and to view the individual permissions, please refer to the citation at the beginning of each chapter. The editor carefully selected each chapter individually to provide a nuanced look at food security and child malnutrition.

Introduction

Food security and child malnutrition are at the forefront of our attention, both nationally and internationally. The articles contained in this compendium include a range of methodologies—literature review, cross-sectional study, longitudinal study, case-control, and even a focus group!—all of which examine this urgent issue, revealing new perspectives and facets of information. Furthermore, this is a not US-centric compendium, but instead includes research into food security measures in other nations around the world. HealthWatch has been a leader in the work being done in this area, and I am particularly happy to be able to include some of their work here. We will first discuss the meaning of food secure versus food insecure, before progressing into the association of food security with nutritional, growth, and physical and mental health outcomes.

—Areej Hassan, MD

The current lack of consensus on the relationships between hunger, malnutrition and food insecurity frustrates efforts to design good policies and programs to deal with the many problems. Disputes over terminology distract from the need for urgent action. Chapter 1 argues that our understanding of food insecurity is incremental: it develops as new research in a variety of food-deprived and nutrition-deprived contexts reveals causes, experiences and consequences and how they are interlinked. If we are to improve beneficiary selection, program targeting and intervention impact assessment, it is vital to coordinate our new understandings. Chapter 1 brings convergence to our understanding of food insecurity by introducing a new framework that visualizes levels of food insecurity, and the concomitant consequences and responses, as a continuum. Some potential benefits of using the continuum as a diagnostic tool are increased focus on less extreme but nevertheless urgent manifestations of food insecurity, more accurate targeting of interventions and better follow-up, and improved accountability for donor spending.

Chapter 2 examines the United States Department of Agriculture's definitions of food security, as well as the measurement and impact of food insecurity. The chapter also explores the history of food insecurity in the United States.

Millions of people in low and low middle income countries suffer from extreme hunger and malnutrition. Research on the effect of food insecurity on child nutrition is concentrated in high income settings and has produced mixed results. Moreover, the existing evidence on food security and nutrition in children in low and middle income countries is either cross-sectional and/ or is based primarily on rural populations. In chapter 3, the authors examine the effect of household food security status and its interaction with household wealth status on stunting among children aged between 6 and 23 months in resource-poor urban setting in Kenya.

The authors use longitudinal data collected between 2006 and 2012 from two informal settlements in Nairobi, Kenya. Mothers and their new-borns were recruited into the study at birth and followed prospectively. The analytical sample comprised 6858 children from 6552 households. Household food security was measured as a latent variable derived from a set of questions capturing the main domains of access, availability and affordability. A composite measure of wealth was calculated using asset ownership and amenities. Nutritional status was measured using Height-for-Age (HFA) z-scores. Children whose HFA z-scores were below −2 standard deviation were categorized as stunted. The authors used Cox regression to analyse the data.

The prevalence of stunting was 49%. The risk of stunting increased by 12% among children from food insecure households. When the joint effect of food security and wealth status was assessed, the risk of stunting increased significantly by 19 and 22% among children from moderately food insecure and severely food insecure households and ranked in the middle poor wealth status. Among the poorest and least poor households, food security was not statistically associated with stunting.

The authors' results shed light on the joint effect of food security and wealth status on stunting. Study findings underscore the need for social protection policies to reduce the high rates of child malnutrition in the urban informal settlements.

Stunting results from decreased food intake, poor diet quality, and a high burden of early childhood infections, and contributes to significant morbidity and mortality worldwide. Although food insecurity is an important determinant of child nutrition, including stunting, development of universal measures has been challenging due to cumbersome nutritional questionnaires and concerns about lack of comparability across populations. The authors of chapter 4 investigate the relationship between household food access, one component of food security, and indicators of nutritional status in early childhood across eight country sites.

The authors administered a socioeconomic survey to 800 households in research sites in eight countries, including a recently validated nine-item food access insecurity questionnaire, and obtained anthropometric measurements from children aged 24 to 60 months. They used multivariable regression models to assess the relationship between household food access insecurity and anthropometry in children and assessed the invariance of that relationship across country sites.

Average age of study children was 41 months. Mean food access insecurity score (range: 0–27) was 5.8, and varied from 2.4 in Nepal to 8.3 in Pakistan. Across sites, the prevalence of stunting (42%) was much higher than the prevalence of wasting (6%). In pooled regression analyses, a 10-point increase in food access insecurity score was associated with a 0.20 SD decrease in height-for-age Z score (95% CI 0.05 to 0.34 SD; p = 0.008). A likelihood ratio test for heterogeneity revealed that this relationship was consistent across countries (p = 0.17).

The study in chapter 4 provides evidence of the validity of using a simple household food access insecurity score to investigate the etiology of childhood growth faltering across diverse geographic settings. Such a measure could be used to direct interventions by identifying children at risk of illness and death related to malnutrition.

Although many studies showed that adolescent food insecurity is a pervasive phenomenon in Southwest Ethiopia, its effect on the linear growth of adolescents has not been documented so far. The study in chapter 5 therefore aimed to longitudinally examine the association between food insecurity and linear growth among adolescents.

Data for this study were obtained from a longitudinal survey of adolescents conducted in Jimma Zone, which followed an initial sample of 2084 randomly selected adolescents aged 13–17 years. The authors used linear mixed effects model for 1431 adolescents who were interviewed in three survey rounds one year apart to compare the effect of food insecurity on linear growth of adolescents.

Overall, 15.9% of the girls and 12.2% of the boys (P=0.018) were food insecure both at baseline and on the year 1 survey, while 5.5% of the girls and 4.4% of the boys (P=0.331) were food insecure in all the three rounds of the survey. In general, a significantly higher proportion of girls (40%) experienced food insecurity at least in one of the survey rounds compared with boys (36.6%) (P=0.045).

The trend of food insecurity showed a very sharp increase over the follow period from the baseline 20.5% to 48.4% on the year 1 survey, which again came down to 27.1% during the year 2 survey.

In the linear mixed effects model, after adjusting for other covariates, the mean height of food insecure girls was shorter by 0.87 cm (P<0.001) compared with food secure girls at baseline. However, during the follow up period on average, the heights of food insecure girls increased by 0.38 cm more per year compared with food secure girls (P<0.066). The mean height of food insecure boys was not significantly different from food secure boys both at baseline and over the follow up period. Over the follow-up period, adolescents who live in rural and semi-urban areas grew significantly more per year than those who live in the urban areas both for girls (P<0.01) and for boys (P<0.01).

Food insecurity is negatively associated with the linear growth of adolescents, especially in girls. High rate of childhood stunting in Ethiopia compounded with lower height of food insecure adolescents compared with their food secure peers calls for the development of direct nutrition interventions targeting adolescents to promote catch-up growth and break the intergenerational cycle of malnutrition.

Chronic malnutrition or stunting among children under 5 years old is affected by several household environmental factors, such as food insecurity, disease burden, and poverty. However, not all children experience stunting even in food insecure conditions. To seek a solution at the local level for preventing stunting, the authors of chapter 6 conducted a cross-sectional study in southeastern Kenya, an area with a high level of food insecurity.

The study was based on a cohort organized to monitor the anthropometric status of children. A structured questionnaire collected information on the following: demographic characteristics, household food security based on the Household Food Insecurity Access Scale (HFIAS), household socioeconomic status (SES), and child health status. The associations between stunting and potential predictors were examined by bivariate and multivariate stepwise logistic regression analyses. Furthermore, analyses stratified by level of food security were conducted to specify factors associated with child stunting in different food insecure groups.

Among 404 children, the prevalence of stunting was 23.3%. The percentage of households with severe food insecurity was 62.5%. In multivariative analysis, there was no statistically significant association with child stunting. However, further analyses conducted separately according to level of food security showed the following significant associations: in the severely food insecure households, feeding tea/porridge with milk (adjusted Odds Ratio [aOR]: 3.22; 95% Confidence Interval [95% CI]: 1.43-7.25); age 2 to 3 years compared with 0 to 5 months old (aOR: 4.04; 95% CI: 1.01-16.14); in households without severe food insecurity, animal rearing (aOR: 3.24; 95% CI: 1.04-10.07); SES with lowest status as reference (aOR range: from 0.13 to 0.22). The number of siblings younger than school age was not significantly associated, but was marginally associated in the latter household group (aOR: 2.81; 95% CI: 0.92-8.58).

The results suggest that measures against childhood stunting should be optimized according to food security level observed in each community.

In a large Canadian study, the authors of chapter 7 examined: (1) the prevalence of hunger due to an inadequate food supply at home; (2) relations between this hunger and a range of health outcomes, and; (3) contextual explanations for any observed associations.

A cross-sectional survey was conducted of 25,912 students aged 11–15 years from 436 Canadian schools. Analyses were descriptive and also involved hierarchical logistic regression models.

Hunger was reported by 25 % of participants, with 4 % reporting this experience "often" or "always". Its prevalence was associated with socio-economic disadvantage and family-related factors, but not with whether or not a student had access to school-based food and nutrition programs. The consistency of hunger's associations with the health outcomes was remarkable. Relations between hunger and health were partially explained when models controlled for family practices, but not the socio-economic or school measures.

Societal responses to hunger certainly require the provision of food, but may also consider family contexts and basic essential elements of care that children need to thrive.

Food insecurity (which can be defined as inadequate access to sufficient, safe, and nutritious food that meets individuals' dietary needs) is concurrently associated with children's psychological difficulties. However, the predictive role of food insecurity with regard to specific types of children's mental health symptoms has not previously been studied. The authors of chapter 8 used data from the Longitudinal Study of Child Development in Québec, LSCDQ, a representative birth cohort study of children born in the Québec region, in Canada, in 1997–1998 (n=2120). Family food insecurity was ascertained when children were 1½ and 4½ years old. Children's mental health symptoms were assessed longitudinally using validated measures of behaviour at ages 4½, 5, 6 and 8 years. Symptom trajectory groups were estimated to identify children with persistently high levels of depression/anxiety (21.0%), aggression (26.2%), and hyperactivity/inattention (6.0%). The prevalence of food insecurity in the study was 5.9%. In sex-adjusted analyses, children from food-insecure families were disproportionately likely to experience persistent symptoms of depression/anxiety (OR: 1.79, 95% CI 1.15–2.79) and hyperactivity/inattention (OR: 3.06, 95% CI 1.68–5.55). After controlling for immigrant status, family structure, maternal age at child's birth, family income, maternal and paternal education, prenatal tobacco exposure, maternal and paternal depression and negative parenting, only persistent hyperactivity/inattention remained associated with food insecurity (fully adjusted OR: 2.65, 95% CI 1.16–6.06). Family food insecurity predicts high levels of children's mental health symptoms, particularly hyperactivity/inattention. Addressing food insecurity and associated problems in families could help reduce the burden of mental health problems in children and reduce social inequalities in development.

Childhood overweight is not restricted to developed countries: a number of lower- and middle-income countries are struggling with the double burden of underweight and overweight. Another public health problem that concerns both developing and, to a lesser extent, developed countries is food insecurity. Chapter 9 presents a comparative gender-based analysis of the association between household food insecurity and overweight among 10-to-11-year-old children living in the Canadian province of Québec and in the country of Jamaica.

Analyses were performed using data from the 2008 round of the Québec Longitudinal Study of Child Development and the Jamaica Youth Risk and Resiliency Behaviour Survey of 2007. Cross-sectional data were obtained from 1190 10-year old children in Québec and 1674 10-11-year-old children in Jamaica. Body mass index was derived using anthropometric measurements and overweight was defined using Cole's age- and sex-specific criteria. Questionnaires were used to collect data on food insecurity. The associations were examined using chi-square tests and multivariate regression models were used to estimate odds ratios (OR) and 95% confidence intervals.

The prevalence of overweight was 26% and 11% ($p < 0.001$) in the Québec and Jamaican samples, respectively. In Québec, the adjusted odds ratio for being overweight was 3.03 (95% CI: 1.8-5.0) among children living in food-insecure households, in comparison to children living in food-secure households. Furthermore, girls who lived in food-insecure households had odds of 4.99 (95% CI: 2.4-10.5) for being overweight in comparison to girls who lived in food-secure households; no such differences were observed among boys. In Jamaica, children who lived in food-insecure households had significantly lower odds (OR 0.65, 95% CI: 0.4-0.9) for being overweight in comparison to children living in food-secure households. No gender differences were observed in the relationship between food-insecurity and overweight/obesity among Jamaican children.

Public health interventions which aim to stem the epidemic of overweight/ obesity should consider gender differences and other family factors associated with overweight/obesity in both developed and developing countries.

Aboriginal children in Canada are at a higher risk for overweight and obesity than other Canadian children. In Northern and remote areas, this has been linked to a lack of affordable nutritious food. However, the majority of Aboriginal children live in urban areas where food choices are more plentiful. Chapter 10 aimed to explore the experiences of food insecurity among Métis and First Nations parents living in urban areas, including the predictors and perceived connections between food insecurity and obesity among Aboriginal children.

Factors influencing children's diets, families' experiences with food insecurity, and coping strategies were explored using focus group discussions with 32 parents and caregivers of Métis and off-reserve First Nations children from Midland-Penetanguishene and London, Ontario. Four focus groups were conducted and transcribed verbatim between July 2011 and March 2013. A thematic analysis was conducted using NVivo software, and second coders ensured reliability of the results.

Caregivers identified low income as an underlying cause of food insecurity within their communities and as contributing to poor nutrition among their children. Families reported a reliance on energy-dense, nutrient-poor foods, as these tended to be more affordable and lasted longer than more nutritious, fresh food options. A lack of transportation also compromised families' ability to purchase healthful food. Aboriginal caregivers also mentioned a lack of access to traditional foods. Coping strategies such as food banks and community programming were not always seen as effective. In fact, some were reported as potentially exacerbating the problem of overweight and obesity among First Nations and Métis children.

Food insecurity manifested itself in different ways, and coping strategies were often insufficient for addressing the lack of fruit and vegetable consumption in Aboriginal children's diets. Results suggest that obesity prevention strategies should take a family-targeted approach that considers the unique barriers facing urban Aboriginal populations. Chapter 10 also reinforces the importance of low income as an important risk factor for obesity among Aboriginal peoples.

America's low-income families struggle to protect their children from multiple threats to their health and growth. Many research and advocacy groups explore the health and educational effects of food insecurity, but less is known about these effects on very young children. Children's HealthWatch, a group of pediatric clinicians and public health researchers, has continuously collected data on the effects of food insecurity alone and in conjunction with other household hardships since 1998. The group's peer reviewed research has shown that a number of economic risks at the household level, including food, housing and energy insecurity, tend to be correlated. These insecurities alone or in conjunction increase the risk that a young child will suffer various negative health consequences, including increases in lifetime hospitalizations, parental report of fair or poor health, or risk for developmental delays. Child food insecurity is an incremental risk indicator above and beyond the risk imposed by household-level food insecurity. The Children's Healthwatch research also suggests public benefits programs modify some of these effects for families experiencing hardships. This empirical evidence is presented in a variety of public venues outside the usual scientific settings, such as congressional hearings, to support the needs of America's most vulnerable population through policy change. Children's HealthWatch research supports legislative solutions to food insecurity, including sustained funding for public programs and re-evaluation of the use of the Thrifty Food Plan as the basis of SNAP benefits calculations. Children's HealthWatch is one of many models to support the American Academy of Pediatrics' call to "stand up, speak up, and step up for children." The authors of chapter 11 argue that no isolated group or single intervention will solve child poverty or multiple hardships. However, working collaboratively each group has a role to play in supporting the health and well-being of young children and their families.

PART I
Defining Food Security

The Food Security Continuum: A Novel Tool for Understanding Food Insecurity as a Range of Experiences

Sheryl L. Hendriks

1.1 A COMPLEX PROBLEM

Food insecurity is a problem with multiple manifestations. Multiple contributing causes—social norms, individual behavior and stages in the human life cycle, food availability and quality—make it a problem requiring comprehensive approaches. The difficulty we face is in bringing convergence to our understanding of the varied experiences of human deprivation so as to improve our response to the problem.

The concept of "food security" first began to attract attention in the 1940s and is now widely used in designing, implementing and evaluating humanitarian emergency and development policies and programs. Today the universal definition of "food security", accepted by the highest level of global governance on food security, the Committee on World Food Security (CFS), describes it as a situation where "all people, at all times, have physical and economic access to sufficient, safe and nutritious food to meet their dietary needs and food preferences for an active healthy life" (CFS 2012 as per the FAO 1996 definition).

However, the usefulness of the concept is constrained by the plurality of ways of understanding the causes and consequences of food insecurity, and the effects of economic, social, political and environmental interventions. Further complicating the issue is the transdisciplinary nature of the food security research field: the experts from different traditional disciplines working together are giving us a more nuanced understanding of the concept but also potentially muddying the waters. Assorted discourses and paradigms compete for domination, leading to conflicts over terms and concepts (Lang and Barling 2012; Candel 2014). The terms "food security", "nutrition security", "food security and nutrition" and "food and nutrition security" are used interchangeably, and some scholars assert a hierarchy among these terms. The proliferation of terms initiated a discussion at the Committee on World Food Security annual meeting in 2012 (CFS 2012). The CFS input note on "coming to terms with terminology" (UNSCN 2012) sets out clearly the origins and development of the contentious terms. But despite a CFS resolution on the use of the terms (CFS 2012), they are still being used interchangeably. This does not make for clarity of understanding or effective policy and program development.

The question of how people experience deprivation continues to perplex us and hamper our efforts to monitor food insecurity situations (Headey and Ecker 2013). Much food security research has attempted to find causal explanations for how material and structural poverty lead to deprivation that manifests in multiple ways. The conclusions often reflect the background and orientation of the researchers. Our plurality of backgrounds (agronomy, economics, sociology, health, nutrition, among others) influences our understanding of what causes food insecurity and consequently of what we must do to deal with it.

The economic, social, environmental and political systems related to food are inextricably inter-connected: eliminating one cause of food insecurity may bring to light a more deeply rooted cause of which the original insecurity may have been a symptom. For example, we might give cash to a poor community to buy food, only to find that lack of cash was a symptom of another problem, such as a lack of local livelihood opportunities. The contributions of different disciplines are needed to deal with multi-layered problems such as this. But theoretical disagreements may distract from the problem. One such disagreement concerns the direction of causality: there is little consensus as to whether food insecurity is a consequence or a predictor of inadequate livelihoods and poor nutrition (Campbell 1991). Pangaribowo et al. (2013) offer a third argument: that food security is an aim in itself, not just a prerequisite for adequate nutrition. This paper argues that the debates lose direction when they fail to differentiate between the risk factors for food insecurity, food insecurity as a phenomenon in itself and the consequences of food insecurity. There seems to be no end to the overlaps and interactions between the categories. Failure to define the topic leads to confusion when it comes to policies and interventions and how to measure their impact.

How we understand and define food insecurity determines how we measure it (Hendriks and Drimie 2011; Coates 2013; Candel 2014). The measurement can take into account quantitative, qualitative, psychological and social or normative constructs of the experience of food insecurity, qualified by their "involuntariness and periodicity" (Campbell 1991, p 410). Competing approaches to food insecurity measurement have emerged over time and no generally accepted framework exists on which to base the measurement. Despite numerous attempts during the 1990s (see Hendriks 2005 and Headey and Ecker 2013 for reviews of these), measuring food insecurity still evades simplification. Each measure both captures and neglects phenomena intrinsic to the concept of food security, thereby subtly creating priorities among food security interventions (Barrett 2010).

Very few measurement systems are based on a full definition of food insecurity. Pinstrup-Andersen (2009: 137) says that if we interpret the FAO definition quoted above "to mean that the nutritional needs of each individual have to be met for the person to be food secure, the FAO estimate of 800 to 900 million under-nourished people would be a gross underestimate of the prevalence of food insecurity". He notes also that "if the estimate of two billion iron deficient people is correct, that number would be the lower bound for the number of food insecure people in the world". He argues that what is at issue is "whether the FAO definition of food security, that is now widely accepted, can be used to disaggregate the concept into different kinds of food insecurity depending on the nature and severity of the problem and the type of solution required".

Understanding the problem of food insecurity is a cumulative process. The following two sections describe how our knowledge has developed incrementally in response to deepening theoretical discourse and also research findings about experiences, causes and consequences. The first of these two sections looks at our incremental theoretical understanding of the four dimensions of food security set out in the World Food Summit definition, availability, accessibility, utilization and stability (FAO 1996), and how these have influenced measurement and interventions. The second discusses how ongoing research has led to an incremental understanding of the experience of human deprivation and the relationships between hunger, under-nutrition, malnutrition and food insecurity. In the next section the author brings together the theoretical and human experience of food security and presents a new framework in which levels of food insecurity are visualized as a continuum. This novel tool combines elements of the triple burden into a single continuum of experiences across emergency and non-emergency as well as obesogenic contexts. The penultimate section discusses some advantages to the application of the continuum for understanding and dealing with food insecurity. The paper concludes by recommending that this diagnostic tool could help improve the accuracy of targeting of interventions, better follow-up and improved accountability for donor spending.

1.2   OUR INCREMENTAL UNDERSTANDING OF THE DIMENSIONS OF FOOD INSECURITY THAT INFLUENCE MEASUREMENT AND INTERVENTION DESIGN

Early conceptualization of food insecurity (prior to the 1980s) relied on a belief that inadequate food supply led to food insecurity. The solution was therefore to produce more food. Consequently, availability of sufficient food was monitored using food balance sheets, from which estimates of food available to meet per capita energy needs were derived (Webb et al. 2006; Pinstrup-Andersen 2009). The physiological consequences of food shortages were measured and monitored anthropometrically. During this period, food security interventions focused on food aid shipments to meet immediate needs and agricultural production strategies to increase food supplies in the long term. But despite increases in global and national food supply following the 1974 world food crisis, under-nutrition rates remained stubbornly high in many parts of the world (Barrett 2010).

The work of Sen in the 1980s led to a widespread awareness that access to food was as essential as having a positive national food stock balance. Sen advanced the understanding of food insecurity when he pointed out that people experience food deprivation because they have difficulty accessing it and not necessarily because it is not available in the marketplace. In his work on poverty Sen viewed food security as a household purchasing power issue affected by access to income and other resources (such as transfers and gifts), market integration, price policies and market conditions (Sen 1981). Food security measurement consequently shifted to identifying subjective experiences of hunger and "coping" strategies as determinants of food security. Consequently, during the 1990s, intervention focus shifted to poverty reduction, food price stabilization and social protection policies (Webb et al. 2006; Barrett 2010).

However, Renzaho and Mellor (2010) warn that it is misleading to measure food security through coping strategies without taking into account the social, cultural, and political contexts in which they occur and that to look at food insecurity solely from the perspective of availability or access to food, without taking into account the importance of how food is used, "paints an incomplete picture". The term "utilization"—one of the four dimensions of food security in the FAO's World Summit 1996 definition—reflects concerns about whether people make good use of the food to which they have access. The concept of utilization, i.e., nutrition, covers dietary quality, especially micronutrient deficiencies, food safety and the ability to absorb and metabolize essential nutrients (Barrett 2010).

It was during the 1990s that the emphasis fell on utilization as the key to attaining food security. Micronutrient deficiencies increase the risk of both chronic and infectious diseases, aggravate the effects of disease and lead to irreversible loss of cognitive and physical function, especially during a child's first 1000 days (from conception to the age of two) (Barrett 2010). Increased awareness of the scale and impact of micronutrient deficiencies led to a new focus on "hidden hunger" and the importance of nutrition-focused interventions to break the cycles of poverty that perpetuate food insecurity. Mere availability of food—at national or household level—does not ensure access to an adequate diet for all citizens. Health and well-being depend on a diverse diet that provides adequate quantities of macro and micro nutrients. Issues of nutritional quality, food safety, access to safe drinking water and sanitation became important in the design of food security programs, with the health sector becoming a major partner in such programs. Nutrition-sensitive and nutrition-specific programs have grown in popularity since the turn of the century. They initially included micronutrient-focused interventions (fortification, supplementation and biofortification) and food-based interventions such as those that support household gardens. The necessity for nutrition-sensitive agricultural interventions became particularly apparent after the global food crisis of 2008/2009 (Frongillo 2013).

Measurement of food security related to utilization is based either on dietary quality (food consumption and dietary diversity) or biochemical analysis of the effects of food consumption. Both are relatively expensive. Moreover, nutrient requirements are individually determined and depend on, among other things, the sex and age of each individual. It is therefore difficult to generalize consumption and nutrition data across populations and the data cannot simply be aggregated at household or national levels as has been done with dietary energy intake in the past (Coates 2013). Such simplification ignores dietary quality. For example, stunting levels of young children can be aggregated at household level and across populations. However, nutrition is only measured at the individual level. Therefore, it cannot be said that a household is well nourished unless all members of the household meet all the criteria for sound nutrition specific to their age, weight, height, sex and level of activity. In the past, energy intake was simply used against referenced standards and thresholds established against standard deviations above or below the norm. Moreover, energy intake is only one requirement for sound nutrition.

These first three food security dimensions—availability, access and utilization—are hierarchical in nature: food availability is necessary but not sufficient for access, and access is necessary but not sufficient for utilization (Webb et al. 2006). However, all three dimensions depend on stable availability, access to food supplies and the resources to acquire adequate food to meet the nutritional needs of all household members throughout their life cycle. To date, very little food security measurement research has focused on the stability dimension of food security, although more recent attention to the concept of resilience may offer measurement and intervention options.

Our expanded knowledge of the link between short-term shocks and long-term development has aroused widespread interest in how people build resilience to adversity (Barrett and Headey 2014). To understand this we need to look at how people cope with and recover from the social, economic and environmental stresses and shocks that lead to hunger and malnutrition (Barrett and Headey 2014). Resilience interventions seek to help households anticipate and deal with stresses, absorb shocks, allocate resources to more profitable enterprises, and improve their chances of escaping poverty (Browne et al. 2014).

Along with increased interest in the concept of resilience, a parallel stream of literature at the turn of the millennium focused on measuring vulnerability (Brown et al. 2014). The terms "vulnerability" and "food insecurity" are often used interchangeably. In order to differentiate them, we should note that food insecurity is a phenomenon whose severity fluctuates, whereas vulnerability is the propensity to fall, or stay, below a food security threshold. In other words, "vulnerability" refers to the ex ante probability of falling or remaining below a specific threshold, while "food insecurity" is the current or ex post measure relative to the threshold (Løvendal and Knowles 2005). However, no standard exists that defines this threshold, and the terms continue to be used loosely, masking the realities of daily deprivation for individuals and communities. Alinovi et al. (2010) argue that the multidimensionality of food security and the unpredictability of shocks make vulnerability measures ineffective, and a lack of longitudinal empirical data on various risks constrains our analysis of trends.

1.3   OUR INCREMENTAL UNDERSTANDING OF THE RELATIONSHIPS BETWEEN HUNGER, UNDER-NUTRITION, MALNUTRITION AND FOOD INSECURITY

Just as our understanding of food security as a concept has followed an incremental development path, so too has our understanding of food insecurity as a lived experience. With time and more research we have come to a better understanding of the ways that various states of deprivation—hunger, under-nutrition, malnutrition and food insecurity—are related. Up to the late 1990s, discussions and research in the field of food security focused on humanitarian crises and famines. However, the last famine in Europe was in the 1940s, in east Asia in the 1960s and in south Asia in the 1970s (Devereux 2009). North Korea faced a famine in 1990 but it was the product of a unique political economy rather than a typical food shortage (Devereux 2009). Four famines in Africa that claimed hundreds of thousands of lives between 1999 and 2012 (Ethiopia, Malawi, Niger and the Horn of Africa) challenged earlier beliefs that famine was primarily related to food shortages. Unlike earlier famines in other parts of the world, these African famines resulted not from a shock (the onset of conflict or a food shortage) but rather from the failure of long-term development processes (Gross and Webb 2006). Even after political stability and economic growth have been restored, the impact of a famine lingers, leaving a nation carrying a burden of lost productivity.

But we do not need to look at the extreme case of a famine to find examples of food deprivation. If we look at developing economies such as Brazil and India, we can see that economies can grow without proportional gains in the nutritional status of the poor (Gross and Webb 2006). Moreover, most deaths in children below the age of five do not happen in acute emergencies—they happen in relatively stable countries (Gross and Webb 2006). Of all food-deprivation-related deaths worldwide in 2004, only 8 % were caused by humanitarian disasters, while 92 % were associated with chronic hunger and malnutrition (Gross and Webb 2006, citing the FAO State of the World Food Security, 2006). The plight of millions of undernourished children in non-emergency zones poses a significant disaster risk unless longer-term coordinated development efforts help avoid disaster (Gross and Webb 2006). Such situations (as was the case in the Niger famine) are a springboard for a sudden leap in mortality when a disaster strikes. Gross and Webb (2006) describe the situation as "a long-running silent emergency" that lays the foundation for future disasters.

Barrett (2010) argues that most severe food insecurity is typically associated with natural and civil disasters. Yet most current food insecurity is not associated with catastrophes but with chronic poverty. Recent attention to development failure helps us understand food insecurity as the consequence of structural poverty and inequality (Hendriks 2013). Structural food insecurity is often the result of extended periods of poverty, lack of assets and inadequate access to productive or financial resources (Pangaribowo et al. 2013). Even in the developed world, hunger is linked to poverty, a situation where there are inadequate resources to obtain food. Poverty is therefore a significant predictor of hunger and food insecurity. People experience food insecurity when they are uncertain about their future supply of and access to food, when their intake (of energy as well as macro and micro nutrients) is inadequate for a healthy life, or when they are obliged to resort to socially unacceptable means of acquiring food. In these situations of food insecurity, hunger and malnutrition are possible, though not necessary, consequences (Frongillo 2013).

The magnitude and ubiquity of such deprivation (across emergency and non-emergency zones) is a significant cause for concern, although the percentage of children who are stunted has been decreasing since 1990. In 2012, 56 % of all stunted children were in Asia and 36 % in Africa, 67 % of all underweight children were in Asia and 29 % in Africa, and 71 % of all severely wasted children were in Asia and 28 % in Africa (UNICEF et al. 2013). Barrett (2010) states that over two billion people worldwide suffer from micronutrient deficiencies—double the number that suffer from inadequate dietary energy. Evidence from many countries shows a weak correlation between energy deprivation and anthropometric indicators of malnutrition—both at the national aggregate and at household levels, emphasizing the importance of overall diet quality (Headey and Ecker 2013). Micronutrient deficiencies increase the risk of both chronic and infectious disease, aggravate the effects of disease, and lead to irreversible loss of cognitive and physical function, especially during the crucial period from 9 to 24 months of age. These irreversible effects foster persistent poverty, thus worsening the consequences of food insecurity.

Prior to the mid-1990s the terms "hunger" and "famine" were frequently used interchangeably (Webb et al. 2006), as were "hunger" and "food insecurity" in the 1980s and 1990s (Campbell 1991). Only in 1999 was the term "food security" used in US empirical assessment tools. Until then, the focus had been on measuring domestic hunger (Wunderlich and Norwood 2006). The change in focus was prompted by the 1984 Report of the President's Task Force on Food Assistance in which it was stated that hunger in the US may not be prolonged enough to manifest in clinical symptoms and affect health (Wunderlich and Norwood 2006). Consequently, hunger in the first world is largely "hidden" and seldom results in overt signs of malnutrition (Riches 1998; Carlson et al. 1999). Both food insecurity and poverty are predictors of nutritional deprivation (Bhattacharya et al. 2004). The term "food insecurity" therefore means more than material deprivation that leads to poverty and more than the presence of hunger; it also covers nutritional deprivation.

However, hunger and malnutrition are possible but not necessary consequences of food insecurity. Differentiating between biological and socioeconomic factors helps us to understand more about the relationship between hunger and malnutrition (Campbell 1991). Te Lintelo et al. (2014: x) define hunger as "the result of an empty stomach" which in turn results from "having insufficient income or social and economic entitlements to access food". Hunger is usually measured in terms of a lack of food—typically as unavailability of food and insufficient energy intake (Masset 2011). Some hunger measures focus on the consequences of hunger—primarily seen as growth faltering and failure, determined through anthropometric measures—but hunger can have other consequences: poor cognitive ability, low productivity, morbidity and mortality (Masset 2011). Some form of under-nutrition is an inevitable consequence of hunger. Consequently, under-nutrition is related to but different from hunger. Under-nutrition can also exist in the absence of hunger: it can be caused by factors unrelated to the quantity of food, such as poor diet quality, or diseases causing malabsorption of nutrients.

Work on understanding famine and HIV/AIDS in Africa in the 1990s has given us a deeper understanding of coping strategies and how households behave when facing hunger (Rugalema 2007). Research has also shown that food needs compete with other needs and that trade-offs involving foods are sometimes made to ensure long-term livelihoods (De Waal and Whiteside 2003; Rugalema 2007). Radimer et al. (1990) identified four aspects common to the experience of food insecurity:

- A quantitative aspect of not having sufficient food
- A qualitative aspect related to the types and diversity of food

- A psychological aspect manifesting as feelings of deprivation or restricted choice and anxiety over food on-hand in the household
- A social or normative aspect in which individuals evaluate their own situation in terms of generally accepted social norms such as the number of meals per day or socially acceptable ways of obtaining food.

Recent work by Frongillo (2013) has further advanced our understanding of the experience of food insecurity. He points out that not all the effects of food insecurity are directly related to food. Worry and anxiety, feelings of alienation, deprivation and distress, and adverse changes in family and social interactions can also lead to poor physical and mental health and weight loss. Understanding the connections between hunger and under-nutrition and these non-food aspects of food insecurity gives us a clearer picture of the complex ways that poverty leads to food insecurity, which in turn leads to poor diet quality and quantity, inadequate nutrition and poor health (Frongillo 2013).

However, hunger and under-nutrition are not the only possible consequences of food insecurity. Since 1995 there has been considerable debate about the link between food insecurity and obesity. The paradox (Caballero 2005) that poverty can make a person obese is being explained now, as we reach a better understanding of the mechanisms of food insecurity. We now understand that poverty is a significant predictor of food insecurity and that food insecurity is a risk factor for poor diets. Until recently, overweight was inevitably blamed on excessive food intake (Townsend et al. 2001). Frongillo (2013) notes that the belief that food insecurity causes only weight loss and not gain is strongly held and often comes with negative sociological and political overtones regarding the reasons why people live in poor conditions. But poverty and food insecurity are both forms of material deprivation that have a range of harmful consequences that could well include excess weight gain (Frongillo 2013).

The notion that there was a relationship between hunger and obesity in the US was first proposed by Dietz (1995: 766), who deduced from his 1994 case study that "food choices or physiologic adaptations in response to episodic food shortages could cause increased body fat". Following this initial awareness, more studies—not only in the developed world, but also in developing countries—showed that adults (especially women) from low income families were more likely to be overweight than those from better-off households (Townsend et al. 2001). Food insecurity-influenced weight gain can be caused by disordered eating patterns. Experiences and fears of food restriction are likely to affect the quality of diet and eating behavior in many ways (Sarlio-Lähteenkorva and

Lahelma 2001). Because a poor household spends a major proportion of its income on food, prices have a strong effect on what foods it selects (Caballero 2005). Globalization of the food system has increased the availability of mass-produced, low-cost, energy-dense and nutrient-poor foods. Because children's nutrient needs are proportionately higher than those of adults, the effect of such foods may be to adversely affect a child's growth but provide sufficient energy for an adult to gain excess weight (Caballero 2005). These effects are not limited to the wealthy; levels of obesity have risen in both developing and developed countries across the world (Stevens et al. 2012; Popkin et al. 2012).

Our new understanding of the way that under-weight and over-weight are related has changed the way we respond to food insecurity. Interventions have shifted from filling the dietary energy gap to improving dietary quality. This demands a broader approach to addressing food insecurity across a spectrum of experiences and outcomes. Availability, access and utilization depend on the broader food system, which in turn depends on the social, economic and political environment. Households are exposed to a range of covariant and idiosyncratic shocks, such as climatic fluctuations, conflict and disease, or job losses and food price increases, that can disrupt food availability, access and utilization (Webb et al. 2006). Interventions therefore need to be very specific and appropriate to the particular context.

Because micronutrient deficiencies reduce well-being and productivity, under-nutrition undermines human capacity and places strain on the state's health and welfare system. We are only now beginning to understand the consequences of an increasing proportion of over-weight people (in both developed and developing countries) in terms of loss of productivity and health care costs. Future food security policies and programs will need to consider the full continuum of food insecurity experiences and consequences if they are to deal with the "triple burden" of hunger, nutrient deficiencies and obesity comprehensively.

1.4   FOOD INSECURITY AS A CONTINUUM

It is internationally recognized that there is no "perfect single measure that captures all aspects of food insecurity" and that food insecurity is not a homogeneous condition easily measured in economic, energy-availability or anthropometric terms (Webb et al. 2006, p1405S). Much food security research since the 1974 global food crisis has focused on understanding the causes of food insecurity in a variety of contexts or developing indices for measuring it.

Yet, after decades of intensive discussion and indicator development, we still do not have a universally accepted food security measurement system that we can apply across emergency and non-emergency contexts and use to develop interventions. One reason for this is the difficulty we experience in getting a grip on all the various strands of the problem. If we are to target our interventions effectively, we need to define the experiences, causes and consequences of food insecurity clearly and understand how the multiple dimensions reinforce each other and compound the problem. Such clarity will help us to predict more accurately who is most likely to be adversely affected by shocks, design more appropriate programs, and determine whether our interventions are working for the intended beneficiaries.

A prerequisite for determining the state of food insecurity is to create a scale against which to measure it. Food insecurity is not a single experience but a sequence of stages reflecting increasing deprivation of basic food needs, accompanied by a process of decision making and behavior in response to increasingly constrained household resources (Rose et al. 1995). It is a continuum of experiences ranging from the most severe form, starvation, to complete food security, defined as a state in which all the criteria of the FAO (1996) definition of food security—" physical and economic access to sufficient, safe and nutritious food to meet ... dietary needs and food preferences for an active healthy life"— are met and there is no worry about future food supply to meet these criteria (Fig. 1). A point to note is that the food (in) security status of an individual or household is not static and can change over time. Many current assessments do not take this into account. It is part of the difficulty in measurement.

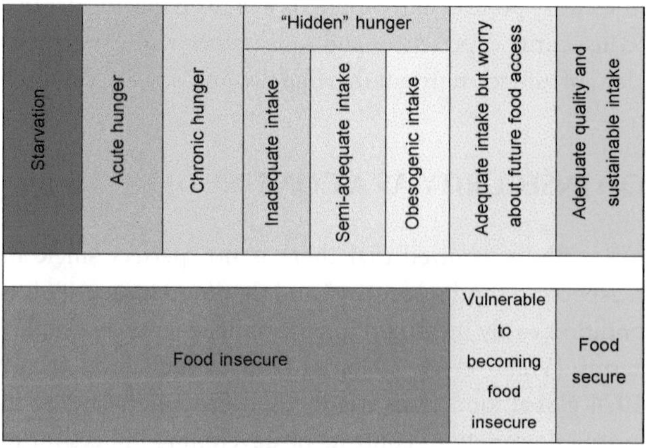

FIGURE 1.1 The food security continuum

Changes in food security status can be temporary, cyclical, medium-term or long-term. These changes may be caused by sudden reductions in the ability to produce or access enough food to maintain the necessary quantity and quality of dietary intake. Food insecurity is usually seasonal or regular (over periods of a month) but may also be aperiodic, i.e., associated with temporary unemployment, episodes of ill health, or other recurring adverse events (Vaitla et al. 2009; Barrett 2010). Such events lead to changes in the food security status of individuals and households and a resultant shifting along the continuum, becoming sometimes more and sometimes less food secure.

Typically, households anticipate such possibilities and routinely take precautions to mitigate their risks. They diversify or increase their options for obtaining food, buffering themselves against shocks that adversely affect or eliminate certain options, or compensating for the loss of one option by replacing it with another. In so doing, they may reduce their risk of more severe food insecurity. However, these traditional ways of coping may erode a household's capacity to withstand shocks and push it further towards food insecurity. Food security interventions should aim not only to save people from dropping back into worse states of food insecurity but to move them along the continuum towards food security and resilience.

Taking what we know about household behavior in response food to shortages (caused by production failure, entitlement failure or inadequate purchasing power), we can identify a continuum of experiences of food insecurity (Fig. 2). Research has shown that the first sign of possible food insecurity is worry over future food supplies or the means to acquire food (Maxwell 1996; Maxwell et al. 1999). If the threat becomes a reality, households start adopting what Barrett (2010, p827) calls "precautionary" strategies.

When the first signs of real food shortages are seen, households find ways of cutting food consumption (Maxwell 1996; Maxwell et al. 1999). These start as subtle changes such as reducing variety, adding ingredients to "stretch" meals (such as bulking up meat dishes with legumes or other vegetables), using cheaper ingredients (such as bones instead of meat) or switching to cheaper foods. Such strategies may compromise the nutritional value of the food. In some cases the strategy is to use fewer processed foods, even though they require more fuel and effort to cook. In other cases it is to consume energy dense "fast foods", if these are easily accessible, as they often cost less than healthy food (Caballero 2005). Another strategy is to skip meals, but choose more energy-dense foods to prevent hunger and consume food in excess when money is again available (Sarlio-Lähteenkorva and Lahelma 2001). Where such practices negatively affect nutritional status, households and individuals will slip further into food insecurity. Subtle consumption reduction and dietary quality compromises may lead to "hidden hunger" as a result of micronutrient deficiencies that are not easily identifiable other than by biochemical analysis. The impact of even small reductions in food and micronutrient intakes can be devastating for the fetus, young children, people whose health and nutritional needs are high (such as pregnant and breast-feeding mothers) and people whose health is already compromised (such as those who are under-weight, malnourished, infirm or elderly). As mentioned above, not all such consumption compromises lead to weight loss. Weight gain that results from a poor diet is "collateral damage — an unintended side effect of hunger itself" (McMillan 2014).

Stage	Starvation	Acute hunger	Chronic hunger	"Hidden" hunger — Inadequate intake	"Hidden" hunger — Semi-adequate intake	"Hidden" hunger — Obesogenic intake	Adequate intake but worry about future food access	Adequate intake with sustainable future supply of food
	Food security							
Classification	Food insecure						Vulnerable to becoming food insecure	Food secure
Characteristic*	Severe wasting (-3SD), Emaciation, oedema, high mortality (especially under	Severe (-2SD) underweight, and /or stunting or oedema or low BMI	Wasting, underweight or Stunting (<1SD) or low BMI	Sub-adequate intake and underweight (between -1SD and normal)	Micro-nutrient deficiencies, seasonal shortages, normal or underweight	Low cost, high carbohydrate and fat intake (BMI over 19/20)	Generally adequate energy intake, normal weight, enjoys dietary diversity	Adequate intake of all nutrients, normal weight, and good dietary diversity
Strategies employed	Household collapse	Sell off productive assets	Sell off non-	Consumption reduction and rationalization	Lack of dietary diversity	Unbalanced diet and perhaps stress eating	Worry about shortages	N/A
	Relience to food insecurity							
Appropriate	Relief interventions: provision of food needs			Mitigation social protection to consumption and consumption			Promotion of sustainable livelihoods	Encouraging the building up of savings, assets draw on in times of shortage

FIGURE 1.2　Continuums of food insecurity, coping strategies and interventions. *Proportion of children six months to five years old who are below 80 % of the median or below -2 Z-score for weight-for-height (wasting), height-for-age (stunting) or weight-for-age (under-weight) (WHO 2010).

At each step towards the insecure end of the continuum, the chances of regaining the former state without assistance are reduced. If food shortages continue or worsen, households will continue cutting portion sizes and skipping meals. They are likely to sell off non-productive assets to buy food, reducing the asset base—an essential element for recovery and resilience (Maxwell 1996)—and heading further in the direction of chronic food insecurity. Continual inadequate intake leads to stunted growth in children and significant productivity losses for all household members. Stunting in early childhood impairs development and limits potential (Alderman 2009). People whose food intake is inadequate are more susceptible to illness, which further compromises health and nutrition. Clinical signs of undernourishment will be evident among the chronically food insecure. At this stage, people need direct access to food to enable them to raise their productive capacity. Chronic food insecurity can only be overcome by long-term development measures to address poverty, such as improved access to productive resources and expanded provision of public services (Pangaribowo et al. 2013). Acute food insecurity is characterized by acute hunger. For people at this point on the continuum, hunger is a daily reality. Households may sell off productive assets to buy food, compromising their future livelihood opportunities and chances of recovery (Maxwell et al. 1999). Here, severe forms of under-nutrition are common, including stunting, wasting and kwashiorkor. Households may resort to reducing household size by sending members to live with relatives (Maxwell et al. 1999). These households need emergency assistance.

Starvation is the extreme experience of food insecurity. When severe hunger is widespread, a famine is declared (Howe and Devereux 2004; Devereux 2009). Extreme manifestations of under-nutrition may appear, such as severe wasting and marasmus. Households may relocate or collapse. Death becomes a possibility, especially for young children.

Classifying the severity of an experience of food insecurity by quantifying the intensity and magnitude of the deprivation is important for creating policies and designing emergency, mitigation and development programs (Howe and Devereux 2004). In Howe and Devereux's famine scale, "severity" refers to the intensity of food insecurity at a particular point in time and "magnitude" to the aggregate impact of the crisis on the affected population. Figure 3 shows a variety of possible scenarios along the food security continuum. Food insecurity may be severe and widespread or severe and individual. Interventions will differ according to the scale and nature of the problem and also according to the availability of the resources required to move individuals and households along the path towards food security.

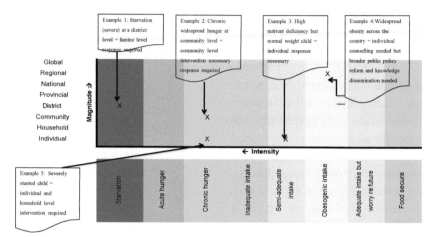

FIGURE 1.3   Continuums of magnitude and intensity of food insecurity

Picturing food insecurity as a continuum makes it clear that realizing the right to food is a progressive process. Various kinds of help can be provided, such as supplying food and ensuring that basic human needs are met, protecting access to food and the means to acquire food and promoting sustainable livelihoods. For households experiencing acute food insecurity or starvation, the priority is to supply food and attend to other needs, such as for water and shelter. The immediate goal of such interventions is to meet the basic needs and alleviate suffering. Once the situation has been stabilized, the aim is to move the beneficiaries to the next stage along the continuum, by providing support to help them recover their livelihoods and assets and to produce or purchase food. Interventions may take many forms, from direct production subsidies to public works programs with food or cash transfers, and can be combined with programs that support adequate consumption. The latter should aim to fill consumption gaps by increasing the opportunity to acquire sufficient food to meet dietary needs. These programs could take many forms, such as food fortification, supplementation, food parcel distribution and school feeding programs.

To ensure a progressive realization of food security, programs need to have clearly defined rules and regulations for beneficiary selection, benefit duration, conditionality (if applicable), exit strategies and monitoring and evaluation. Clear targets must be set, with measurable impact indicators. Such indicators should measure improvement in the food security continuum stages. For a program to be sustainable, and the goal of long-term national food security to be achieved, program managers and beneficiaries must be given incentives to move progressively towards food security.

1.5   ADVANTAGES OF THE CONTINUUM

The food security continuum introduced in this paper brings together many aspects of food insecurity: the FAO's four dimensions (availability, accessibility, utilization and stability), nutritional inadequacy, the triple burden of hunger, nutrient deficiencies and obesity. It provides a comprehensive approach to understanding the experience and consequences of food insecurity and thus a basis for identifying food insecure individuals and households and designing programs appropriate to their situation. It makes it possible to identify individuals and households at various stages of food insecurity and estimate the severity of their problem. By showing us who they are and how many, it enables more accurate targeting of beneficiaries. This means that scarce resources can be used more efficiently. The continuum helps us to see the link between what we know of the experience of food insecurity and how it makes people behave (their coping strategies) and the typical symptoms they exhibit as a consequence of these strategies. It helps us to focus on each specific situation, taking into account differences in resource bases, livelihoods and individual or household decision-making. Its first big advantage is that it enables us to sidestep the complications introduced by theoretical disagreements about causality and interrelatedness and move more directly to acting to help the victims. A second advantage of the continuum is that it provides concrete characterization of the affected individuals and households. We position victims at the various stages along the continuum according to universal quantitative measurements related to food security, such as population referenced anthropometric measures, and also according to their context, noting that coping strategies and asset bases are specific to communities and populations. By thus increasing accuracy, the continuum should reduce targeting errors (both inclusion and exclusion errors).

The third advantage is that it enables us not only to design interventions appropriate to the stage that the victims have reached but also to monitor the interventions effectively. The specific indicators identified for each stage along the continuum (at individual or household level, depending on the purpose of the intervention and its targeted beneficiaries) can be traced over time. Because a variety of indicators are possible for each stage, the selection of indicators can be determined by what data is collected regularly and adapted to rapid appraisal frameworks for emergency situations or to more impact-focused long-term monitoring and evaluation indicators. It would be possible to integrate the continuum indicators into the post-2015 Development Goals as it seems the Sustainable Development Goals may include aspects of both hunger and poverty along with acknowledgement that individual nutritional adequacy is the foundation for achieving food security.

1.6 CONCLUSION

As observed in the introduction to this paper, understanding food insecurity requires inputs from different disciplines, but we should not allow academic disagreements to distract us from finding practical solutions. We should not waste time haggling over definitions and terminology and arguing about causes. We need a sound framework, based on the experiences and consequences of food insecurity that integrates the components of adequate food consumption, dietary quality relevant to the life cycle of each person and sustainable livelihoods to ensure future food security. While the food security continuum presented in this paper does not specify indicators, it offers a visual guide for more concerted effort to identify food insecurity in comparable ways across populations and monitor the course of interventions.

The food security continuum builds on our iterative understanding of food insecurity as a phenomenon. It categorizes levels of intensity of food insecurity and matches them with appropriate interventions at each stage. It brings convergence to the economic, social, environmental and political aspects of food insecurity and, by focusing on individual experience, it considers the right to food. It is a step towards designing appropriate policies and programs to respond to the plight of deprived individuals, households and communities. It can help us achieve the two essential goals of any program: first to attend to people's immediate needs, and second to help them build resilience in the face of stresses and shocks. It is a progressive, rights-based approach to food security, intended to help us move beneficiaries along the path towards food security.

Until recently, many famine interventions were initiated in response to the proportion of the population experiencing extreme starvation over a prolonged period on a scale that could not be ignored (Howe and Devereux 2004). The continuum is not meant to replace existing famine early warning systems or food security monitoring systems but rather to extend such efforts beyond relief operations towards a more integrated understanding of food security across the range of experiences. We must not wait until a food shortage becomes a significant humanitarian crisis before acting. The prevalence and scale of hunger and malnutrition worldwide is unacceptable. It requires a comprehensive approach that can assist national governments to achieve global development goals.

The continuum draws our attention to the less extreme manifestations of food insecurity that demand our ongoing rather than emergency attention. It enables us to visualize the triple burden of hunger, nutrient deficiencies and obesity in a comprehensive way. It provides a framework for focusing policy attention on the entire food system and anticipating the outcome of interventions and policies. Applying this comprehensive approach across the full range of experiences may help us avoid some of the unintended consequences of food security interventions such as the consumption changes that may accompany increased incomes in societies with easy access to cheap "obesogenic" foods (Pincock 2011) that encourage excessive weight gain.

To deal with all the stages along the food insecurity continuum demands a multi-sectoral commitment to working together with communities to realize their right to food and formulate food security action plans. Governments must provide a bundle of public goods to support progressive steps towards long-term household food security. In enabling us to measure and monitor food insecurity at different levels and thus improve targeting and intervention design, the continuum will also improve accountability for public and donor spending.

REFERENCES

1. Alderman, H. (2009). The economic cost of a poor start to life. Journal of Developmental Origins of Health and Disease, 1(1), 19–25.
2. Alinovi, L., Mane, E., & Romano, D. (2010). Measuring household resilience to food insecurity: An application to Palestinian households. In R. Benedetti, M. Bee, G. Espa, & F. Piersimoni (Eds.), Agricultural survey methods. Chichester: Wiley.
3. Barrett, C. B. (2010). Measuring food insecurity. Science, 327, 825. doi:10.1126/science.1182768.
4. Barrett, C. B., & Headey, D. (2014). Measuring resilience in a risky world: Why, where, how and who? 2020 Conference Brief 1: Building Resilience for Food and Nutrition Security. Washington, DC: IFPRI (International Food Policy Research Institute).
5. Bhattacharya, J., Currie, J., & Haider, S. (2004). Poverty, food insecurity, and nutritional outcomes in children and adults. Journal of Health Economics, 23, 839–862.
6. Browne, M., Ortmann, G. F., & Hendriks, S. L. (2014). Developing a resilience indicator for food security monitoring and evaluation. Agrekon, 53(2), 25–46.
7. Caballero, B. (2005). A nutrition paradox: underweight and obesity in developing countries. New England Journal of Medicine, 352(15), 1515–1516.
8. Campbell, C. C. (1991). Food security: a nutritional outcome of a predictor variable? Journal of Nutrition, 121, 408–415.

9. Candel, J. L. (2014). Food security governance: a systemic literature review. Food Security, 6, 585–601.

10. Carlson, S. J., Andrews, M. S., & Bickel, G. W. (1999). Measuring food insecurity and hunger in the United States: development of a national benchmark measure and prevalence estimates. Journal of Nutrition, 1129, 2. doi:10.1371/journal.pmed.1000101.

11. CFS (Committee on World Food Security). (2012). Report of the 39th session of the Committee on World Food Security (CFS), Rome, 15–20 October 2012. Rome: CFS.

12. Coates, J. (2013). Build it back better: deconstructing food security for improved measurement and action. Global Food Security, 2, 188–194.

13. De Waal, A., & Whiteside, A. (2003). New variant famine: AIDS and food crisis in southern Africa. Lancet, 362(9391), 1234–7.

14. Devereux, S. (2009). Why does famine persist in Africa? Food Security, 1, 25–35.

15. Dietz, W. H. (1995). Does hunger cause obesity? Pediatrics, 95, 766.

16. FAO (Food and Agriculture Organization). (1996). World food summit: Rome declaration on world food security. Rome: FAO.

17. Frongillo, E. A. (2013). Confronting myths about household food insecurity and excess weight. Cadernos de Saúde Pública, 29(2), 229–230.

18. Gross, R., & Webb, P. (2006). Wasting time for wasted children: severe child under-nutrition must be resolved in non-emergency settings. The Lancet, 367(9517), 1209–1211. doi:10.1016/S0140-6736(06)68509-7.

19. Headey, D., & Ecker, O. (2013). Rethinking the measurement of food security: from first principles to best practice. Food Security, 5, 327–343.

20. Hendriks, S. L. (2005). The challenges facing empirical estimation of food (in) security in South Africa. Development Southern Africa, 22(1), 103–123.

21. Hendriks, S. L. (2013). Will renewed attention and investment in African agriculture ensure sound nutrition? European Journal of Development Research, 25, 36–43.

22. Hendriks, S. L., & Drimie, S. (2011). Chapter 7, global food crisis and African response: Lessons for emergency response planning. In D. S. Miller & J. S. Rivera (Eds.), Comparative emergency management: Examining global and regional responses to disasters (pp. 153–173). Boca Raton: CRC/Taylor & Francis.

23. Howe, P., & Devereux, S. (2004). Famine intensity and magnitude scales: a proposal for an instrumental definition of famine. Disasters, 28(4), 353–373.

24. Lang, T., & Barling, D. (2012). Food security and food sustainability: reformulating the debate. Geographical Journal, 178(4), 313–326.

25. Løvendal, C. R., & Knowles, M. (2005). Tomorrow's hunger: A framework for analyzing vulnerability to food insecurity. Agriculture and Development Economics Division ESA working paper, 05–07. Rome: Food and Agriculture Organization of the United Nations.

26. Masset, E. (2011). A review of hunger indexes and methods to monitor country commitment to fighting hunger. Food Policy, 36, S102–S108.

27. Maxwell, D. G. (1996). Measuring food insecurity: the frequency and severity of "coping strategies". Food Policy, 21(3), 291–303.

28. Maxwell, D., Ahiadeke, C., Levin, C., Armar-Klemesu, M., Zakariah, S., & Lamptey, G. M. (1999). Alternative food-security indicators: revisiting the frequency and severity of "coping strategies". Food Policy, 24, 411–429.

29. McMillan, T. (2014). The new face of hunger: Why are people malnourished in the richest country on Earth? National Geographic, August 2014. www.nationalgeographic.com/foodfeatures/hunger/. Accessed 28 August 2014.

30. Pangaribowo, E. H, Gerber, N., & Torero, M. (2013). Food and nutrition security indicators: A review. Working paper no. 108. Zentrum für Entwicklungsforschung (ZEF) Working Paper Series, Department of Political and Cultural Change, Center for Development Research, University of Bonn.

31. Pincock, S. (2011). Boyd Swinburn: combating obesity at the community level. Lancet, 378(9793), 761. doi:10.1016/S0140-6736(11)61364-0.

32. Pinstrup-Andersen, P. (2009). Food security: definition and measurement. Food Security, 1, 5–7.

33. Popkin, B. M., Adair, L. S., & Ng, S. W. (2012). Now and then: The global nutrition transition: the pandemic of obesity in developing countries. Nutrition Review, 70(1), 3–21. doi:10.1111/j.1753-4887.2011.00456.x.

34. Radimer, K. L., Olson, C. M., & Campbell, C. C. (1990). Development of indicators to assess hunger. Journal of Nutrition, 120, 1544–1548.

35. Renzaho, A. M. N., & Mellor, D. (2010). Food security measurement in cultural pluralism: missing the point or conceptual misunderstanding? Nutrition, 26, 1–9.

36. Riches, G. (1998). First world hunger: Food security and welfare politics. New York: Palgrave Macmillan.

37. Rose, D., Basiotis, P. P., & Klein, B. W. (1995). Improving federal efforts to assess hunger and food insecurity. Food Review, 18, 18.

38. Rugalema, G. (2007). Coping or struggling? a journey into the impact of HIV/AIDS in southern Africa. Review of African Political Economy, 27(86), 537–545. doi:10.1080/03056240008704488.

39. Sarlio-Lähteenkorva, S., & Lahelma, E. (2001). Food insecurity is associated with past and present economic disadvantage and body mass index. Journal of Nutrition, 1(131), 2880–2884.

40. Sen, A. (1981). Poverty and famines: An essay on entitlement and deprivation. Oxford: Clarendon.

41. Stevens, G. A., Singh, G. M., Lu, Y., Danaei, G., Lin, J. K., Finucane, M. M., Bahalim, A. N., McIntire, R. K., Gutierrez, H. R., Cowan, M., Paciorek, C. J., Farzadfar, F., Riley, L., Ezzati, M., & the Global Burden of Metabolic Risk Factors of Chronic Diseases Collaborating Group (Body Mass Index). (2012). National, regional, and global trends in adult overweight and obesity prevalence. Population Health Metrics, 10, 22. doi:10.1186/1478-7954-10-22.

42. Te Lintelo, D. J. H., Haddad, L. J., Lakshman, R., & Gatellier, K. (2014). The Hunger and Nutrition Commitment Index (HANCI 2013): Measuring the political commitment to reduce hunger and under nutrition in developing countries. Brighton: Institute for Development Studies, University of Sussex.

43. Townsend, M. S., Peerson, J., Love, B., Achterberg, C., & Murphy, S. P. (2001). Food insecurity is positively related to overweight in women. Journal of Nutrition, 131(6), 1738–1745.

44. UNICEF, WHO & World Bank (United Nations' Children's Fund, World Health Organization & World Bank). (2013). Joint UNICEF—WHO – The World Bank Child Malnutrition Database: Estimates for 2012 and launch of interactive data dashboards. www.who.int/nutgrowthdb/jme_2012_summary_note_v2.pdf?ua=1. Accessed 11 September 2014.

45. UNSCN (United Nations Standing Committee on Nutrition). (2012). Coming to terms with terminology: Food security, nutrition security, food security and nutrition, food and nutrition security. Rome: CFS (Committee on World Food Security). www.fao.org/fsnforum/sites/default/files/file/Terminology/MD776(CFS____Coming_to_terms_with_Terminology).pdf. Accessed 26 August 2014.
46. Vaitla, B., Devereux, S., & Swan, S. H. (2009). Seasonal hunger: a neglected problem with proven solutions. PLoS Medicine, 6(6), e1000101.
47. CrossRefPubMedCentralPubMed
48. Webb, P., Coates, J., Frongillo, E. A., Lorge Rogers, B., Swindale, A., & Bilinsky, P. (2006). Measuring household food insecurity: why it's so important and yet so difficult to do. Journal of Nutrition, 136, 1404S–1408S.
49. WHO (World Health Organization). (2010). Nutrition landscape information system: Country profile indicators. Interpretation guide. Geneva: WHO.
50. Wunderlich, G. S., & Norwood, J. L. (2006). Food insecurity and hunger in the United States: An assessment of the measure. Washington, DC: Panel to Review the US Department of Agriculture's Measurement of Food Insecurity and Hunger, Committee on National Statistics, Division of Behavioral and Social Sciences and Education, National Research Council of the National Academies of Science. National Academies Press.

CHAPTER 2

USDA Definition of Food Security in the U.S.

United States Department of Agriculture

2.1 OVERVIEW

Food security means access by all people at all times to enough food for an active, healthy life.

ERS plays a leading role in Federal research on food security and food security measurement in U.S. households and communities and provides data access and technical support to social science scholars to facilitate their research on food security. ERS research focuses on:

- food security in U.S. households,
- food security's impact on the well-being of children, adults, families, and communities, and
- food security's relationship to public policies, public assistance programs, and the economy.

2.2 DEFINITIONS OF FOOD SECURITY

2.2.1 Ranges of Food Security and Food Insecurity

In 2006, USDA introduced new language to describe ranges of severity of food insecurity. USDA made these changes in response to recommendations by an expert panel convened at USDA's request by the Committee on National

United States Department of Agriculture Economic Research Service. Available online at http://www.ers.usda.gov/ topics/food-nutrition-assistance/food-security-in-the-us.aspx.

Statistics (CNSTAT) of the National Academies. Even though new labels were introduced, the methods used to assess households' food security remained unchanged, so statistics for 2005 and later years are directly comparable with those for earlier years for the corresponding categories.

2.2.1.1 USDA's Labels Describe Ranges of Food Security

2.2.1.1.1 Food Security

- High food security (old label=Food security): no reported indications of food-access problems or limitations.
- Marginal food security (old label=Food security): one or two reported indications—typically of anxiety over food sufficiency or shortage of food in the house. Little or no indication of changes in diets or food intake.

2.2.1.1.2 Food Insecurity

- Low food security (old label=Food insecurity without hunger): reports of reduced quality, variety, or desirability of diet. Little or no indication of reduced food intake.
- Very low food security (old label=Food insecurity with hunger): Reports of multiple indications of disrupted eating patterns and reduced food intake.

2.2.2 CNSTAT Review and Recommendations

USDA requested the review by CNSTAT to ensure that the measurement methods USDA uses to assess households' access—or lack of access—to adequate food and the language used to describe those conditions are conceptually and operationally sound and that they convey useful and relevant information to policy officials and the public. The panel convened by CNSTAT to conduct this study included economists, sociologists, nutritionists, statisticians, and other researchers. One of the central issues the CNSTAT panel addressed was whether the concepts and definitions underlying the measurement methods—especially the concept and definition of hunger and the relationship between hunger and food insecurity—were appropriate for the policy context in which food security statistics are used.

The CNSTAT panel:

- Recommended that USDA continue to measure and monitor food insecurity regularly in a household survey.
- Affirmed the appropriateness of the general methodology currently used to measure food insecurity.
- Suggested several ways in which the methodology might be refined (contingent on confirmatory research). ERS has recently published Assessing Potential Technical Enhancements to the U.S. Household Food Security Measures and is continuing to conduct research on these issues.

The CNSTAT panel also recommended that USDA make a clear and explicit distinction between food insecurity and hunger.

- Food insecurity—the condition assessed in the food security survey and represented in USDA food security reports—is a household-level economic and social condition of limited or uncertain access to adequate food.
- Hunger is an individual-level physiological condition that may result from food insecurity.

The word "hunger," the panel stated in its final report, "...should refer to a potential consequence of food insecurity that, because of prolonged, involuntary lack of food, results in discomfort, illness, weakness, or pain that goes beyond the usual uneasy sensation." To measure hunger in this sense would require collection of more detailed and extensive information on physiological experiences of individual household members than could be accomplished effectively in the context of the CPS. The panel recommended, therefore, that new methods be developed to measure hunger and that a national assessment of hunger be conducted using an appropriate survey of individuals rather than a survey of households.

The CNSTAT panel also recommended that USDA consider alternative labels to convey the severity of food insecurity without using the word "hunger," since hunger is not adequately assessed in the food security survey. USDA concurred with this recommendation and, accordingly, introduced the new labels "low food security" and "very low food security" in 2006.

2.2.3   Characteristics of Households with Very Low Food Security

Conditions reported by households with very low food security are compared with those reported by food-secure households and by households with low (but not very low) food security in the following graph:

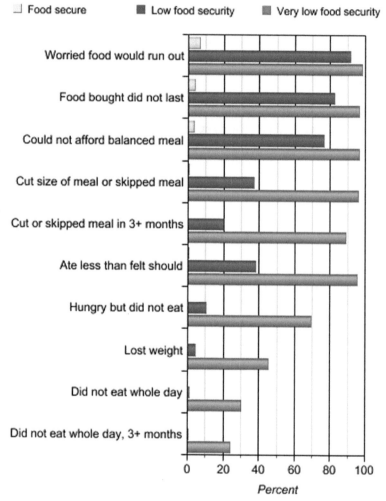

FIGURE 2.1   Percentage of households reporting indicators of adult food insecurity, by food security status, 2014.

Source: Calculated by ERS using data from the December 2014 Current Population Survey Food Security Supplement.

The defining characteristic of very low food security is that, at times during the year, the food intake of household members is reduced and their normal eating patterns are disrupted because the household lacks money and other resources for food. Very low food security can be characterized in terms of the conditions that households in this category typically report in the annual food security survey.

- 98 percent reported having worried that their food would run out before they got money to buy more.
- 97 percent reported that the food they bought just did not last, and they did not have money to get more.
- 97 percent reported that they could not afford to eat balanced meals.
- 96 percent reported that an adult had cut the size of meals or skipped meals because there was not enough money for food.
- 89 percent reported that this had occurred in 3 or more months.
- 96 percent of respondents reported that they had eaten less than they felt they should because there was not enough money for food.
- 69 percent of respondents reported that they had been hungry but did not eat because they could not afford enough food.
- 45 percent of respondents reported having lost weight because they did not have enough money for food.
- 30 percent reported that an adult did not eat for a whole day because there was not enough money for food.
- 24 percent reported that this had occurred in 3 or more months.

All households without children that were classified as having very low food security reported at least six of these conditions, and 69 percent reported seven or more. Food-insecure conditions in households with children followed a similar pattern.

2.3   KEY STATISTICS & GRAPHICS

2.3.1   Food Security Status of U.S. Households in 2014

Food secure—These households had access, at all times, to enough food for an active, healthy life for all household members.

- 86.0 percent (106.6 million) of U.S. households were food secure throughout 2014.
- Essentially unchanged from 85.7 percent in 2013.

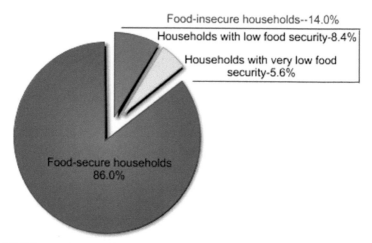

Food-insecure households--14.0%

Households with low food security-8.4%

Households with very low food security-5.6%

Food-secure households 86.0%

FIGURE 2.2   U.S. households by food security status, 2014.

Source: Calculated by ERS using data from the December 2014 Current Population Survey Food Security Supplement.

Food insecure—At times during the year, these households were uncertain of having, or unable to acquire, enough food to meet the needs of all their members because they had insufficient money or other resources for food. Food-insecure households include those with low food security and very low food security.

- 14.0 percent (17.4 million) of U.S. households were food insecure at some time during 2014.
- Essentially unchanged from 14.3 percent in 2013.

Low food security—These food-insecure households obtained enough food to avoid substantially disrupting their eating patterns or reducing food intake by using a variety of coping strategies, such as eating less varied diets, participating in Federal food assistance programs, or getting emergency food from community food pantries.

- 8.4 percent (10.5 million) of U.S. households had low food security in 2014.
- Essentially unchanged from 8.7 percent in 2013.

Very low food security—In these food-insecure households, normal eating patterns of one or more household members were disrupted and food intake was reduced at times during the year because they had insufficient money or other resources for food.

- 5.6 percent (6.9 million) of U.S. households had very low food security at some time during 2014.
- Unchanged from 5.6 percent in 2013.

2.3.2 Food Security Status of U.S. Households with Children in 2014

Among U.S. households with children under age 18:

- 80.8 percent were food secure in 2014.
- In 9.8 percent of households with children, only adults were food insecure.
- Both children and adults were food insecure in 9.4 percent of households with children (3.7 million households).
- Although children are usually protected from substantial reductions in food intake even in households with very low food security, nevertheless, in about 1.1 percent of households with children (422,000 households), one or more child also experienced reduced food intake and disrupted eating patterns at some time during the year.

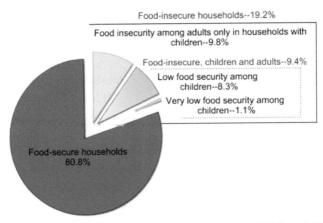

FIGURE 2.3   U.S. households with children by food security status of adults and children, 2014.

Source: Calculated by ERS using data from the December 2014 Current Population Survey Food Security Supplement.

2.3.3   How Many People Lived in Food-Insecure Households?

In 2014:

- 48.1 million people lived in food-insecure households.
- 12.4 million adults lived in households with very low food security.
- 7.9 million children lived in food-insecure households in which children, along with adults, were food insecure.
- 914,000 children (1.2 percent of the Nation's children) lived in households in which one or more child experienced very low food security.

2.3.4   Food Insecurity by Household Characteristics

The prevalence of food insecurity varied considerably among household types. Rates of food insecurity were higher than the national average (14.0 percent) for the following groups:

- All households with children (19.2 percent),
- Households with children under age 6 (19.9 percent),
- Households with children headed by a single woman (35.3 percent),
- Households with children headed by a single man (21.7 percent),
- Black, non-Hispanic households (26.1 percent),
- Hispanic households (22.4 percent), and
- Low-income households with incomes below 185 percent of the poverty threshold (33.7 percent; the Federal poverty line was $24,008 for a family of four in 2014).

Overall, households with children had a substantially higher rate of food insecurity (19.2 percent) than those without children (11.7 percent). Among households with children, married-couple families had the lowest rate of food insecurity (12.4 percent).

The prevalence of food insecurity was highest for households located in nonmetropolitan areas (17.1 percent), intermediate for those in principal cities of metropolitan areas (15.7 percent), and lowest in suburban and other metropolitan areas outside principal cities (11.8 percent).

Regionally, the food insecurity rate was higher in the South (15.1 percent) than in the Northeast (13.3 percent), Midwest (13.8 percent), and West (13.1 percent).

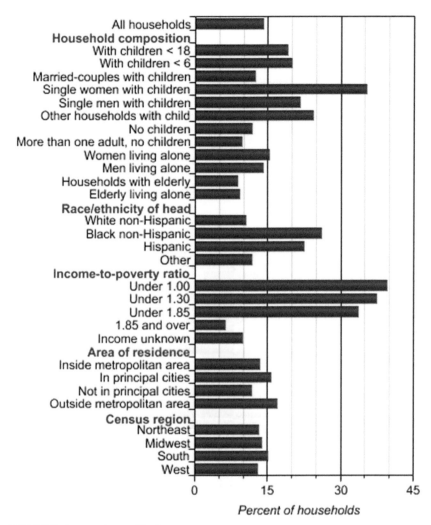

FIGURE 2.4 Prevalence of food insecurity, 2014.

Source: Calculated by ERS using data from the December 2014 Current Population Survey Food Security Supplement.

2.3.4 Very Low Food Security by Household Characteristics

The prevalence of very low food security in various types of households followed a pattern similar to that observed for food insecurity overall. Very low food security was more prevalent than the national average (5.6 percent) for the following groups:

- Households with children headed by a single woman (12.8 percent) or a single man (7.0 percent),
- Women living alone and men living alone (7.2 percent each),
- Black, non-Hispanic households (10.4 percent),
- Hispanic households (6.9 percent),
- Households with incomes below 185 percent of the poverty line (14.5 percent), and
- Households located outside metropolitan areas (7.3 percent).

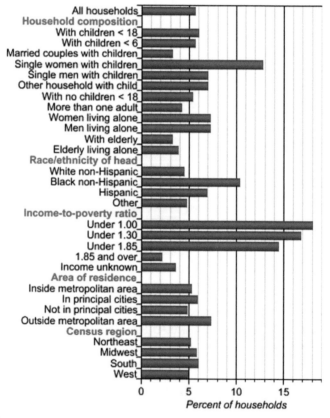

FIGURE 2.5   Prevalence of very low food security, 2014.

Source: Calculated by ERS using data from the December 2014 Current Population Survey Food Security Supplement.

2.3.5   Trends in Prevalence Rates

The prevalence of food insecurity was essentially unchanged from 2013 to 2014 and from 2012 to 2014. That is, the changes were within the range that could have resulted from sampling variation. The cumulative decline from 2011 (14.9 percent) to 2014 (14.0 percent) was statistically significant. Over the previous decade, food insecurity increased from 10.5 percent in 2000 to nearly 12 percent in 2004, declined to 11 percent in 2005-07, then increased in 2008 (14.6 percent), remaining essentially unchanged at that level in 2009 and 2010.

The prevalence of very low food security was essentially unchanged from 2011 and 2012 (5.7 percent in both years) to 2013 and 2014 (5.6 percent in both years). The prevalence of very low food security was also 5.7 percent in 2008 and 2009. In 2010, the prevalence of very low food security had declined to 5.4 percent. Prior to 2008, the prevalence of very low food security had increased from 3.1 percent in 2000 to 3.9 percent in 2004, and remained essentially unchanged through 2007.

The year-to-year deviations from a consistent downward trend between 1995 and 2000 include a substantial 2-year cycle that is believed to result from seasonal effects on food security prevalence rates. The CPS food security surveys over this period were conducted in April in odd-numbered years and August or September in even-numbered years. Measured prevalence of food insecurity was higher in the August/September collections, suggesting a seasonal-response effect. In 2001 and later years, the surveys were conducted in early December, which avoids seasonal effects in interpreting annual changes.

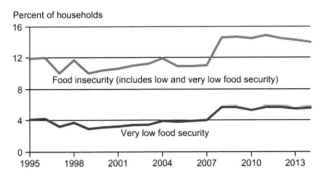

FIGURE 2.6   Trends in prevalence rates of food insecurity and very low food security in U.S. households, 1995-2014. Prevalence rates for 1996 and 1997 were adjusted for the estimated effects of differences in data collection screening protocols used in those years.

Source: Calculated by ERS based on Current Population Survey Food Security Supplement data.

2.3.5   State-Level Prevalence of Food Insecurity

Prevalence rates of food insecurity varied considerably from State to State. Data for 3 years, 2012-14, were combined to provide more reliable statistics at the State level. Estimated prevalence rates of food insecurity during this 3-year period ranged from 8.4 percent in North Dakota to 22.0 percent in Mississippi; estimated prevalence rates of very low food security ranged from 2.9 percent in North Dakota to 8.1 percent in Arkansas.

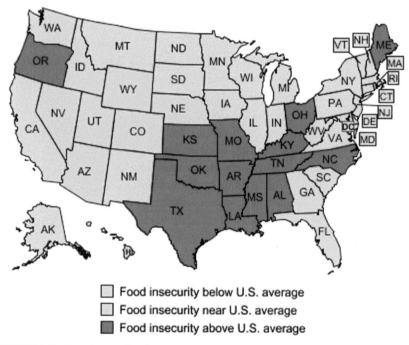

FIGURE 2.7   Prevalence of food insecurity, average 2012-2014.

Source: Calculated by ERS using data from the December 2014 Current Population Survey Food Security Supplement.

2.4   FREQUENCY OF FOOD INSECURITY

The U.S. Household Food Security Scale is designed to register even occasional or episodic occurrences of food insecurity. Some households may be classified as food insecure or as having very low food security based on a single episode during the year. A more complete picture of the temporal patterns of food insecurity in U.S. households sheds light on the nature and seriousness of the food access problems households face and can aid in the design and management of programs to improve food security.

2.4.1   Frequency of Food Insecurity During the Year

ERS analyzed responses to questions in the food security survey about how frequently various food-insecure conditions occurred during the year, whether they occurred during the 30 days prior to the survey, and, if so, for how many days. Findings include:

- About one-fourth of households with very low food security at any time during the year experienced it rarely or occasionally-in only 1 or 2 months of the year. For three-fourths, very low food security recurred in 3 or more months of the year.
- For about one-fourth of food-insecure households and one-third of those with very low food security, the occurrence was frequent or chronic.
- On average, households that were food insecure at some time during the year were food insecure in 7 months during the year.
- On average, households with very low food security at some time during the year experienced it in 7 months during the year and in 1 to 7 days in each of those months.

2.4.2   Prevalence of Food Insecurity and very Low Food Security, by Reference Period

Prevalence rates of food insecurity and very low food security during the 30 days preceding the food security survey were considerably lower than the annual rates. Some households were food insecure only early in the year but not in the 30 days prior to the survey interview. The estimated prevalence of very low food security during a single day was lower yet—between 0.7 and 1.1 percent of households. The daily prevalence rate probably is biased considerably downward due to the omission of homeless people from the survey, which is based on household addresses.

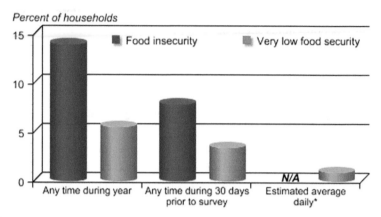

FIGURE 2.8   Prevalence of food insecurity and very low food security, by reference period, 2014.

N/A = Estimated average daily occurrence of food insecurity is not available because information was not collected on the number of days that less severe food-insecure conditions occurred.
*Estimated average daily prevalence of very low food security is between 0.7 and 1.1 percent of households.
Source: Calculated by ERS using data from the December 2014 Current Population Survey Food Security Supplement.

2.4.3   Frequency of Food Insecurity During a 5-Year Period

The food security survey which is the basis for USDA's annual food security statistics measures food insecurity for 2 time periods—1) during the previous year and 2) during the previous 30 days. However, knowing how often and how long households are food insecure over longer time periods is important for understanding the extent and character of food insecurity and for maximizing the effectiveness of programs aimed at alleviating it. Two studies commissioned by ERS found spells of food insecurity to be generally of short duration (see "Food Insecurity in U.S. Households Rarely Persists Over Many Years"). For example, one study found that half of households that were food insecure at some time during the 5-year study period experienced the condition in just a single year, and only 6 percent were food insecure in all 5 years. However, the fact that households move in and out of food insecurity also means that a considerably larger number of households experience food insecurity at some time over a period of several years than in any single year.

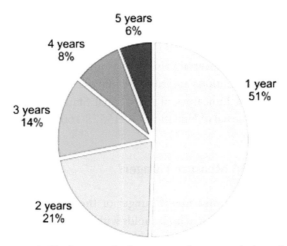

FIGURE 2.9 Households that were food insecure at least once during a 5-year period, by number of years of food insecurity.

Source: USDA, Economic Research Service summary of findings from a study by Parke E. Wilde et al. published in the *Journal of Hunger and Environmental Nutrition*.

2.5 MEASUREMENT

This section provides an overview of how household food security and food insecurity are measured. For detailed technical information on measurement methods, questionnaires, and calculating food security scales, see Food Security in the U.S.: Survey Tools.

2.5.1 What is Food Security?

Food security for a household means access by all members at all times to enough food for an active, healthy life. Food security includes at a minimum:

- The ready availability of nutritionally adequate and safe foods.
- Assured ability to acquire acceptable foods in socially acceptable ways (that is, without resorting to emergency food supplies, scavenging, stealing, or other coping strategies).

2.5.2   ...and Food Insecurity?

Food insecurity is limited or uncertain availability of nutritionally adequate and safe foods or limited or uncertain ability to acquire acceptable foods in socially acceptable ways. (Definitions are from the Life Sciences Research Office, S.A. Andersen, ed., "Core Indicators of Nutritional State for Difficult to Sample Populations," The Journal of Nutrition 120:1557S-1600S, 1990.)

2.5.3   Does USDA Measure Hunger?

USDA does not have a measure of hunger or the number of hungry people. Prior to 2006, USDA described households with very low food security as "food insecure with hunger" and characterized them as households in which one or more people were hungry at times during the year because they could not afford enough food. "Hunger" in that description referred to "the uneasy or painful sensation caused by lack of food."

In 2006, USDA introduced the new description "very low food security" to replace "food insecurity with hunger," recognizing more explicitly that, although hunger is related to food insecurity, it is a different phenomenon. Food insecurity is a household-level economic and social condition of limited access to food, while hunger is an individual-level physiological condition that may result from food insecurity.

Information about the incidence of hunger is of considerable interest and potential value for policy and program design. But providing precise and useful information about hunger is hampered by lack of a consistent meaning of the word. "Hunger" is understood variously by different people to refer to conditions across a broad range of severity, from rather mild food insecurity to prolonged clinical undernutrition.

USDA sought guidance from the Committee on National Statistics (CNSTAT) of the National Academies on the use of the word "hunger" in connection with food insecurity. The independent panel of experts convened by CNSTAT concluded that in official statistics, resource-constrained hunger (i.e., physiological hunger resulting from food insecurity) "...should refer to a potential consequence of food insecurity that, because of prolonged, involuntary lack of food, results in discomfort, illness, weakness, or pain that goes beyond the usual uneasy sensation."

Validated methods have not yet been developed to measure resource-constrained hunger in this sense, in the context of U.S. conditions. Such measurement would require collection of more detailed and extensive information on physiological experiences of individual household members than could be accomplished effectively in the context of USDA's annual household food security survey.

USDA's measurement of food insecurity, then, provides some information about the economic and social contexts that may lead to hunger but does not assess the extent to which hunger actually ensues.

2.5.4 How are Food Security and Insecurity Measured?

The food security status of each household lies somewhere along a continuum extending from high food security to very low food security. This continuum is divided into four ranges, characterized as follows:

1. High food security—Households had no problems, or anxiety about, consistently accessing adequate food.
2. Marginal food security—Households had problems at times, or anxiety about, accessing adequate food, but the quality, variety, and quantity of their food intake were not substantially reduced.
3. Low food security—Households reduced the quality, variety, and desirability of their diets, but the quantity of food intake and normal eating patterns were not substantially disrupted.
4. Very low food security—At times during the year, eating patterns of one or more household members were disrupted and food intake reduced because the household lacked money and other resources for food.

USDA introduced the above labels for ranges of food security in 2006. See Food Security in the U.S.: Definitions of Food Security for further information.

For most reporting purposes, USDA describes households with high or marginal food security as food secure and those with low or very low food security as food insecure.

Placement on this continuum is determined by the household's responses to a series of questions about behaviors and experiences associated with difficulty in meeting food needs. The questions cover a wide range of severity of food insecurity.

- Least severe: Was this statement often, sometimes, or never true for you in the last 12 months? "We worried whether our food would run out before we got money to buy more."
- Somewhat more severe: Was this statement often, sometimes, or never true for you in the last 12 months? "We couldn't afford to eat balanced meals."
- Midrange severity: In the last 12 months, did you ever cut the size of your meals or skip meals because there wasn't enough money for food?
- Most severe: In the last 12 months, did you ever not eat for a whole day because there wasn't enough money for food?

In the last 12 months, did any of the children ever not eat for a whole day because there wasn't enough money for food?

Every question specifies the period (last 12 months) and specifies lack of resources as the reason for the behavior or experience ("we couldn't afford more food," "there was not enough money for food.")

2.5.4.1   Food Insecure

Households that report three or more conditions that indicate food insecurity are classified as "food insecure." That is, they were at times unable to acquire adequate food for one or more household members because they had insufficient money and other resources for food. The three least severe conditions that would result in a household being classified as food insecure are:

- They worried whether their food would run out before they got money to buy more.
- The food they bought didn't last, and they didn't have money to get more.
- They couldn't afford to eat balanced meals.

Households are also classified as food insecure if they report any combination of three or more conditions, including any more severe conditions.

2.5.4.2   Very Low Food Security

Households having "very low food security" were food insecure to the extent that eating patterns of one or more household members were disrupted and their food intake reduced, at least some time during the year, because they could not afford enough food. To be classified as having "very low food security," households with no children present must report at least the three conditions listed above and also that:

- Adults ate less than they felt they should.
- Adults cut the size of meals or skipped meals and did so in 3 or more months.

Many report additional, more severe experiences and behaviors as well. If there are children in the household, their experiences and behaviors are also assessed, and an additional two affirmative responses are required for a classification of very low food security.

2.5.5 Survey Questions Used by USDA to Assess Household Food Security

1. "We worried whether our food would run out before we got money to buy more." Was that often, sometimes, or never true for you in the last 12 months?
2. "The food that we bought just didn't last and we didn't have money to get more." Was that often, sometimes, or never true for you in the last 12 months?
3. "We couldn't afford to eat balanced meals." Was that often, sometimes, or never true for you in the last 12 months?
4. In the last 12 months, did you or other adults in the household ever cut the size of your meals or skip meals because there wasn't enough money for food? (Yes/No)
5. (If yes to question 4) How often did this happen--almost every month, some months but not every month, or in only 1 or 2 months?
6. In the last 12 months, did you ever eat less than you felt you should because there wasn't enough money for food? (Yes/No)
7. In the last 12 months, were you ever hungry, but didn't eat, because there wasn't enough money for food? (Yes/No)
8. In the last 12 months, did you lose weight because there wasn't enough money for food? (Yes/No)
9. In the last 12 months did you or other adults in your household ever not eat for a whole day because there wasn't enough money for food? (Yes/No)

10. (If yes to question 9) How often did this happen--almost every month, some months but not every month, or in only 1 or 2 months?

(Questions 11-18 were asked only if the household included children age 0-17)

11. "We relied on only a few kinds of low-cost food to feed our children because we were running out of money to buy food." Was that often, sometimes, or never true for you in the last 12 months?

12. "We couldn't feed our children a balanced meal, because we couldn't afford that." Was that often, sometimes, or never true for you in the last 12 months?

13. "The children were not eating enough because we just couldn't afford enough food." Was that often, sometimes, or never true for you in the last 12 months?

14. In the last 12 months, did you ever cut the size of any of the children's meals because there wasn't enough money for food? (Yes/No)

15. In the last 12 months, were the children ever hungry but you just couldn't afford more food? (Yes/No)

16. In the last 12 months, did any of the children ever skip a meal because there wasn't enough money for food? (Yes/No)

17. (If yes to question 16) How often did this happen--almost every month, some months but not every month, or in only 1 or 2 months?

18. In the last 12 months did any of the children ever not eat for a whole day because there wasn't enough money for food? (Yes/No)

2.5.6 How Many Households are Interviewed in the National Food Security Surveys?

USDA's food security statistics are based on a national food security survey conducted as an annual supplement to the monthly Current Population Survey (CPS). The CPS is a nationally representative survey conducted by the Census Bureau for the Bureau of Labor Statistics. The CPS provides data for the Nation's monthly unemployment statistics and annual income and poverty statistics.

In December of each year, after completing the labor force interview, about 45,000 households respond to the food security questions and to questions about food spending and about the use of Federal and community food assistance programs. The households interviewed in the CPS are selected to be representative of all civilian households at State and national levels.

2.6   HISTORY & BACKGROUND

2.6.1   Early History

The food security statistics reported by ERS are based on a survey measure developed by the U.S. Food Security Measurement Project, an ongoing collaboration among Federal agencies, academic researchers, and private commercial and nonprofit organizations. The measure was developed in response to the National Nutrition Monitoring and Related Research Act of 1990 (NNMRR).

The Ten-Year Comprehensive Plan developed under that Act specified the following task: "Recommend a standardized mechanism and instrument(s) for defining and obtaining data on the prevalence of 'food insecurity' or 'food insufficiency' in the United States and methodologies that can be used across the NNMRR Program and at State and local levels."

Beginning in 1992, USDA staff reviewed the existing research literature on the conceptual basis for measuring food insecurity and on the practical problems of developing a survey instrument for use in sample surveys at national, State, and local levels.

In January 1994, USDA's Food and Nutrition Service (FNS) joined with the U.S. Department of Health and Human Services' National Center for Health Statistics to sponsor a National Conference on Food Security Measurement and Research. The conference brought together leading academic experts, private researchers, and key staff of the concerned Federal agencies. The conference identified the appropriate conceptual basis for a national measure of food insecurity. The conference also reached a working agreement as to the best operational form for implementing such a measure in national surveys.

2.6.2   CPS Food Security Supplement

The U.S. Census Bureau carried out a cognitive assessment and field test of the food security questionnaire. They finalized the questionnaire and administered it as a supplement to the Current Population Survey (CPS) of April 1995.

The Food Security Supplement was repeated again in September 1996, April 1997, August 1998, April 1999, September 2000, April and December 2001, and annually in December since 2001. Minor modifications to the questionnaire format and screening procedures were made over the first several years, and a more substantial revision in screening and format, designed to reduce respondent burden and improve data quality, was introduced with the August 1998 survey. However, the content of the 18 questions upon which the U.S. Food Security Scale is based remained constant in all years.

2.6.3   Development of the Household Food Security Scale

Initial analysis of the 1995 data in *Household Food Security in the United States in 1995: Technical Report of the Food Security Measurement Project* was conducted by Abt Associates Inc. through a cooperative venture with FNS, an interagency working group on food security measurement, and other key researchers involved in developing the questionnaire. The Abt team used nonlinear factor analysis and other state-of-the-art statistical methods to produce a scale that measures the severity of deprivation in basic food needs as experienced by U.S. households. Extensive testing established the validity and reliability of the scale and its applicability across various household types in the broad national sample.

Following collection of the September 1996 and April 1997 CPS food security data, Mathematica Policy Research, Inc. (MPR), under a contract awarded by FNS, independently reproduced the results from the 1995 CPS food security data, estimated prevalence rates of food insecurity for 1996 and 1997, and assessed the stability and robustness of the measurement model when applied to the separate datasets. The MPR findings in *Household Food Security in the United States, 1995-1997: Technical Issues and Statistical Report* established the stability of the food security measure over the 1995-97 period. That is, the relative severities of the items were found to be nearly invariant across years and across major population groups and household types.

2.6.4   ERS Sponsors the Food Security Survey

In 1998, the Economic Research Service (ERS) assumed sponsorship of the Census Bureau's annual food security survey and responsibility for analyzing and reporting the data and for coordinating ongoing USDA research on food security and food security measurement.

ERS collaborated with MPR and FNS to develop and finalize standardized procedures for calculating the household food security scale and analyzed the data from 1998 and later years using these procedures. ERS and IQ Solutions analyzed data from the 1998 and 1999 surveys, found that the scale continued to be stable, and examined additional technical measurement and estimation issues (see Household Food Security in the United States, 1998 and 1999: Technical Report).

2.6.5 Committee on National Statistics Reviews the Food Security Measure

In 2003-06 an expert panel convened by the Committee on National Statistics (CNSTAT) of the National Academies conducted a thorough review of the food security measurement methods. USDA requested the review to ensure that the measurement methods USDA uses to assess households' access—and lack of access—to adequate food and the language used to describe those conditions are scientifically sound and that they convey useful and relevant information to policy officials and the public.

The panel convened by CNSTAT to conduct this study included economists, sociologists, nutritionists, statisticians, and other researchers. Two of the central issues the CNSTAT panel addressed were:

- Are the concept and definition of hunger appropriate for the policy context in which food security statistics are used?
- Is the relationship between hunger and food insecurity appropriately represented in the language used to report food security statistics?

The CNSTAT panel recommended that USDA continue to measure and monitor food insecurity regularly in a household survey, affirmed the appropriateness of the general methodology currently used to measure food insecurity, and suggested several ways in which the methodology might be refined (contingent on confirmatory research).

The CNSTAT panel recommended that USDA make a clear and explicit distinction between food insecurity and hunger and consider alternative labels to convey the severity of food insecurity without using the word "hunger." USDA concurred with this recommendation and, accordingly, introduced the new labels "low food security" and "very low food security" to replace "food insecurity without hunger" and "food insecurity with hunger," respectively.

USDA collaborated with partners in the food security measurement community to explore how best to implement other recommendations of the CNSTAT panel. In December 2012, ERS published a technical bulletin describing findings from assessments of five potential technical enhancements to the statistical methods used by USDA to measure food security (see Assessing Potential Technical Enhancements to the U.S. Household Food Security Measures).

2.6.6   Other Surveys Collect Food Security Data

The Federal food security measurement project has developed standardized questionnaires and methods for editing and scoring to produce household summary measures of food security status. These modules are now in use in several national surveys including:

- Survey of Program Dynamics (SPD).
- National Health and Nutrition Examination Survey (NHANES IV).
- National Center for Educational Statistics' Early Childhood Longitudinal Study-Kindergarten Cohort (ECLS-K).
- National Center for Educational Statistics' Early Childhood Longitudinal Study-Birth Cohort (ECLS-B).
- National Health Interview Survey (NHIS).
- Panel Study of Income Dynamics (PSID).
- Survey of Income and Program Participation (SIPP).
- A growing number of State, local, and regional studies.

2.7   COMMUNITY FOOD SECURITY

Community food security has roots in disciplines such as community nutrition, nutrition education, public health, sustainable agriculture, and anti-hunger and community development. There is no universally accepted definition of community food security. In the broadest terms, community food security can be described as a prevention-oriented concept that supports the development and enhancement of sustainable, community-based strategies:

- To improve access of low-income households to healthful nutritious food supplies.
- To increase the self-reliance of communities in providing for their own food needs.
- To promote comprehensive responses to local food, farm, and nutrition issues.

Policies and programs implemented under the label of community food security address a diverse range of issues, including:

- Food availability and affordability.
- Direct food marketing.
- Diet-related health problems.
- Participation in and access to Federal nutrition assistance programs.
- Ecologically sustainable agricultural production.
- Farmland preservation.
- Economic viability of rural communities.
- Economic opportunity and job security.
- Community development and social cohesion.

2.7.1   Recent ERS Research

Local Food Systems: Concepts, Impacts, and Issues—This comprehensive overview of local food systems explores alternative definitions of local food, estimates market size and reach, describes the characteristics of local consumers and producers, and examines early indications of the economic and health impacts of local food systems. Statistics suggest that local food markets account for a small, but growing, share of U.S. agricultural production. For smaller farms, direct marketing to consumers accounts for a higher percentage of their sales than for larger farms.

Food Environment Atlas—Food environment factors—such as store/restaurant proximity, food prices, food and nutrition assistance programs, and community characteristics—interact to influence food choices and diet quality. The Food Environment Atlas assembles statistics on food environment indicators to stimulate research on the determinants of food choices and diet quality and provides a spatial overview of a community's ability to access healthy food and its success in doing so. The Atlas includes indicators of the food environment in three broad categories—food choices, health and well-being, and community characteristics.

Access to Affordable and Nutritious Food: Updated Estimates of Distance to Supermarkets Using 2010 Data—Efforts to encourage Americans to improve their diets and to eat more nutritious foods presume that a wide variety of these foods are accessible to everyone. But for some Americans and in some communities, access to healthy foods may be limited. Using population data from the 2010 Census, income and vehicle availability data from the 2006-2010

American Community Survey, and a 2010 directory of supermarkets, this report estimates that 9.7 percent of the U.S. population, or 29.7 million people, live in low-income areas more than 1 mile from a supermarket. However, only 1.8 percent of all households live more than 1 mile from a supermarket and do not have a vehicle. Estimated distance to the nearest three supermarkets is an indicator of the choices available to consumers and the level of competition among stores. Estimates show that half of the U.S. population lives within 2 miles of three supermarkets.

2.7.1.1 Examples of Strategies and Activities

- Farmers' markets that boost incomes of small local farmers and increase consumers' access to fresh produce.
- Community-supported agriculture programs that provide small-scale farmers with economic stability while ensuring consumer members high-quality produce, often at below retail prices.
- Farm-to-school initiatives that help local farmers sell fresh fruits and vegetables directly to school meals programs.
- Supplemental Nutrition Assistance Program (SNAP) outreach programs that help increase the number of eligible households that participate in the Supplemental Nutrition Assistance Program.

PART II

Food Security, Nutrition, and Growth and Development

Household Food (In)Security and Nutritional Status of Urban Poor Children Aged 6 to 23 Months in Kenya

Maurice Mutisya, Ngianga-Bakwin Kandala,
Moses Waithanji Ngware, and
Caroline W. Kabiru

3.1 BACKGROUND

A vast pool of evidence shows that food security is associated with a number of human and economic development outcomes [1, 2]. In light of the high burden of malnutrition and its consequences, the Sustainable Development Goals (SDGs) highlight food security as a human right that needs to be addressed with urgency [3]. Despite this recognition, millions of people in low and low middle income countries suffer from extreme hunger and malnutrition [1]. Household food insecurity is associated with poor nutritional health [2, 4]. Among children, poor nutritional status has negative consequences on growth and development, especially during the early years of life [5]. While poor nutrition status in children includes over nutrition, it often refers to cases of undernutrition [6]. Undernutrition refers to deficiency of protein energy, micronutrients and vitamins as well as minerals essential for growth.

Globally, there has been a decline in malnutrition levels from the 1990s; however, the levels in sub Saharan Africa have remained high [7, 8]. Close to 90 % of stunted (a long term measure of malnutrition) children in the world live in Africa and Asia, with the prevalence of stunting in Africa being 36 % in 2011 [9]. In Kenya the prevalence of stunting was 26 % in 2014 [10]. In urban poor settings in low and middle income countries where few households can produce their own food, the prevalence of stunting may be even higher. In informal settlements in Nairobi, for example, 60 % of children below 5 years were stunted in 2010 as compared to 17 % for the whole of Nairobi [10, 11].

Food security and nutrition are different concepts that are intricately linked resulting to some researchers to apply the two concepts interchangeably. However, food security is a means to nutritional status, and is necessary but not sufficient for nutrition [12]. There exists an extensive body of literature on nutritional status among under-five children and women [1, 13]. The focus on children is because their physiology, growth and development are sensitive to both adequate food (food secure) and nutrition [11, 14, 15]. Further, childhood malnutrition contributes to nearly one third of under-five deaths in the world and up to 11 % of Disability Adjusted Life Years (DALYS), with 80 % of the deaths occurring in low income countries [13].

The first 1000 days of a child life (from conception to the second birthday) have been noted to be very crucial [16, 17]. This period is characterized by rapid brain growth [18]. Therefore, any disruptions, especially occasioned by malnutrition, during this period can have both short and long term effects on education, health and productivity [8].

Research in high income countries shows that food insecurity is associated with poor health outcomes across the population [19, 20]. A study of eight low income countries found food insecurity to be associated with low height-for-age (stunting) Z-scores [21]. In Canada, food insufficiency was found to be associated with poor self-reported health status [20]. This highlights the importance of food security as a determinant of individual physical, social and mental wellbeing.

Research on the association between food insecurity and malnutrition has produced mixed results. While some studies have found a positive relationship [14, 22, 23] others have found no association or even a negative one [24]. Moreover, the existing evidence on food security and nutrition in children in low and middle income countries is either cross-sectional and/or is based primarily on rural populations. Using longitudinal data collected between 2006 and 2012, we model the relationship between food insecurity and nutrition (measured by stunting) controlling for other covariates among children aged between 6 and 23 months in two urban informal settlements in Nairobi, Kenya. Fotso et al. [11] drew on the same dataset to analyse the effect of poverty on child growth using multi-level modelling. The main outcome was stunting measured by z-scores. Poverty status was measured using several indicators including asset index, household expenditure, food security index and self-reported poverty (based on a subjective index). Overall, the food security index was associated with child stunting for ages 6 to 11 months. The household asset index was also a strong predictor of stunting, and the effect increased with increased age of the child. The study however, modelled the different poverty indicators separately/ independently. By so doing, they assumed the different poverty indicators affect stunting in isolation. In addition, the effect of food insecurity on children is hypothesised to take place from the point of introduction to complementary feeding, that is, from 6 months, yet in their study they included all children from birth (age 0). Moreover, as a longitudinal study, which was subject to attrition, it was unusual to use a multi-level model. This model does not take into consideration the loss of follow-up and the time amount of time those lost to follow-up have contributed (exposure duration) to the study, which may have resulted in an underestimate of the effect of the poverty measures on child nutrition.

To address the limitations of the Fotso et al. [11] study, in the current study we used survival analysis, which takes care of the exposure period, hence reducing the bias due to attrition. As food security, a proximate determinant of child nutrition, is likely to be strongly influenced by poverty [13], we interacted the asset wealth index with food security status in order to establish whether the effect of food security differs by the levels of asset wealth status. We therefore hypothesise that 1) household food security is associated with the nutrition status of children aged between 6 and 23 months; and 2) the effect of household food security on stunting does not vary by household wealth status, a proxy measure of poverty.

3.2 METHODS

3.2.1 Study Setting

The study was conducted in two informal settlements—Korogocho and Viwandani—located in Nairobi, Kenya. The two study sites are part of the Nairobi Urban Health and Demographic Surveillance System (NUHDSS). The NUHDSS was initiated in 2002 to collect health and demographic statistics from an urban poor population. From 2003, the NUHDSS framework has provided opportunities for nesting studies, including the current study. For detailed description of the NUHDSS see Beguy et al. [25].

3.2.2   Data and Data Source

Data for this study come from the Maternal and Child Health (MCH) study (2006–2010), which was a sub-study of the broader Urbanization, Poverty and Health Dynamics project, and the INDEPTH Vaccination Project (IVP) study (2011 – 2013). The latter was a continuation of the MCH study. The MCH study was nested within the NUHDSS framework. The project targeted all women of reproductive health residing in the two study communities who gave birth between the duration of study—2006 to 2013. Under the MCH project, mothers and their new-borns were recruited upon delivery. The mothers and their children were then followed prospectively until the child was 5 years or until when they exited from the study either through death or out migration. Data were collected on the mother's social demographic characteristics, her health seeking behaviour during and after delivery, feeding practices, immunization of the child as well as the anthropometric measures for both the child and mother. Upon recruitment, three follow-up visits, in this study referred to as updates, were made each calendar year. The following variables were extracted from two data sets: 1) Child characteristics that include date of birth, date of recruitment and subsequent visits, gender of the child, immunization, anthropometric measures, and birth weight and; 2) maternal characteristics that included the mother age at birth, parity, education level and health seeking behaviour. By 2013, 7452 children had been recruited to the study. During analysis, we excluded children with missing information on stunting between the ages 6 and 23 as well as those who were lost to follow-up before they attained the age of 6 months. The final sample consisted of 6858 children contributing to 101,686 person months.

3.2.3   Variables and Measurement

The dependent variable is stunting, which is Height for Age (HFA). Stunting is used here because it is a measure of long term food deprivation (chronic malnutrition) and illness making it a good indicator of child nutrition [26]. We calculated z-scores for the HFA using the 'WHO Child Growth Charts and WHO Reference 2007 Charts' for children aged up to 2 years. This was suitable because analysis was restricted to children aged between 6 and 24 months. The entry age was set at 6 months, which marks the end of exclusive breastfeeding and introduction to complimentary feeding. The Z-scores show the number of standard deviations of a child on a particular anthropometric measure in relation to a mean or median value. In this regard, those with z-scores of 2 standard deviations of height for age below the WHO reference median were categorized as stunted. Those with a score of above 2 standard deviations were categorized as normal (not stunted) [27]. Child anthropometric measures were obtained during each visit and therefore, stunting was calculated at the each points of visit.

The primary independent variable was household food security status. Food security exists "when all people at all times have access to sufficient, safe, nutritious food to maintain a healthy and active life" [28]. Food security status was computed from a set of questions that captured the domains of food access as described in Radimer framework [29]. The questions assessed the frequency in the 30 days preceding the survey with which households: did not have adequate food; were worried about food availability; lacked enough money to purchase food; and children and adults had to forgo food for a whole day because there was not enough food. The response were coded as either '0 = never true', '1 = sometimes true' and '2 = often true.' The respondent to the food security component was the household head who in his or her absence, the spouse or someone who had enough information and was credible enough was interviewed. Responses were recoded into binary responses: 'often true' were coded as '1' and the rest '0' and as described by [30]. We tested for agreement between the items and found a Cronbach's Alpha of 0.72, indicating a good item reliability [31]. A composite score was generated by summing the items and categorized as 1 = food secure (score of 0); 2 = moderate food insecure (score of 1 or 2); and 3 = severely food insecure (score of more than 2).

The second independent variable was the household asset wealth index, a latent variable computed from a composite measure of household assets and amenities. Principal Component Analysis (PCA) was used to reduce the multidimensional nature of the data to a single score that was categorized into three groups: Poorest, middle poor and least poor [32].

3.2.4 Statistical Analysis

Data were managed and analysed in STATA 13.1. Both descriptive and inferential statistics were used for analysis. Frequencies and percentages were computed to describe the key socio-demographic characteristics of the study sample. In addition, descriptive statistics were used to estimate the prevalence of stunting in the sample. As multiple measures on stunting exist for each child, the exposure, which is the age of the child, was calculated for each visit. We used Cox regression models to estimate the survival time from age six to first stunting and to assess whether the survival time significantly varied by household food security status. The Cox regression models allowed us to control for other known determinants of stunting. In our study we restricted analysis to time to the first stunting. We tested the assumption of proportional hazard in the Cox regression, which is that the hazards are constant between the food security status and wealth status categories being compared. To test this assumption, we used Kaplan-Meier Curves and the log rank test. We also tested the assumption by interacting survival time with time varying covariate. Different Cox regression models were fitted: 1) unadjusted models with the key independent variables that included food security and household; 2) adjusted Cox regression with two main covariates—food security and wealth index; 3) a fully adjusted model, including all the covariates; and 4) a fully adjusted model with all covariates and the interaction between wealth index (poorest, middle poor and least poor) and food security status. The latter model was used to determine whether the effect of food security on stunting was the same across the wealth quintiles.

For the Cox regression model, age in months was the main dependent variable with a dummy variable indicating whether the child is stunted or not. Each child was observed from birth between 2006 and 2013 until either the child was stunted, was censored due to loss of follow-up, out-migration or end of the follow-up for the child who aged above 23 months.

3.2.5   Ethical Clearance and Informed Consent

Ethical clearance for both the MCH and IVP studies were granted by the Kenya Medical Research Institute (KEMRI). In addition, ethical clearance to use the data for secondary analyses was obtained from the University of the Witwatersrand, Human Research Ethics Committee and AMREF Kenya. Informed consent was obtained from all individual participants included in the study. All procedures were conducted in accordance with the ethical standards of the institutional and/or national research committee and with the 1964 Helsinki declaration and its later amendments or comparable ethical standards.

3.3   RESULTS

Table 1 presents the background characteristics of the study sample at the point of entry into the study (about age of 6 months). The table also shows the proportion of stunted children for each variable category. Overall, the prevalence of stunting among children aged between 6 and 23 months in the study areas was about 49 %. The study sample consisted of nearly an equal number of male and female children, however, the proportion of stunted male children (54 %) was higher than females (44 %). Although a slightly higher proportion of children lived in Korogocho (53 %) than Viwandani, a greater proportion of children in Viwandani (52 %) were stunted compared with Korogocho (45 %).

TABLE 3.1   Background characteristics of the study sample at entry and levels of stunting (n = 6858)

Characteristic	Number		Percentage	
	Total	**Stunted**	**Sample**	**Stunted**
Overall	6858	3349	-	48.83
Child sex**				
Male	3462	1858	50.48	53.67
Female	3396	1491	49.52	43.90
Food security**				
Food secure	1930	823	28.14	42.64
Moderate	3432	1708	50.04	49.77
Food insecure	1496	818	21.81	54.68
Wealth index**				
Poorest	2778	1466	40.51	52.77
Middle	2125	970	30.99	45.65
Least poor	1955	913	28.51	46.70
Mother education**				
Incomplete primary/no education	1902	991	27.73	52.10
Completed primary	3251	1621	47.40	49.86
Secondary plus	1705	737	24.86	43.23
Birth weight**				
Below 2500	346	166	5.05	47.98
2500 - 2900	1007	548	14.68	54.42
= > 3000	3817	1795	55.66	47.03
No birth weight record	1688	840	24.61	49.76

TABLE 3.1 *(Continued)*

Characteristic	Number		Percentage	
	Total	**Stunted**	**Sample**	**Stunted**
Breast feeding				
Yes	72	41	1.05	56.94
Introduced to foods	6786	3308	98.95	48.75
Parity*				
1	2097	962	30.58	45.88
2	2016	982	29.40	48.71
3	1227	606	17.89	49.39
4	683	346	9.96	50.66
5 plus	835	453	12.18	54.25
Study site**				
Korogocho	3613	1894	52.68	52.42
Viwandani	3245	1455	47.32	44.84
HHH Education**				
No education	291	151	4.24	51.89
Primary	4172	2117	60.83	50.74
Secondary & above	2393	1081	34.92	45.14
HHH sex				
Female	1606	797	23.42	49.63
Male	5225	2552	76.58	48.59
Mean mother age[a]	6558		25.04 (5.92)	24.73(5.86)
Mean HHH age[a]	6558		34.49 (9.65)	33.92 (9.63)
Average HH size[a]	6558		4.67 (1.98)	4.64 (1.90)

Significant at *$p < 0.05$; **$p < 0.01$ when testing difference in the proportion of children stunted by each variables; HH = Household; HHH = HH head; aMean and standard deviations reported

Two key variables were time variant—food security and household asset wealth index. The two variables were calculated for all the households in the two study sites and thereafter merged with the data used in this analysis. At entry, 50 % of children were from moderately food insecure households, while 22 % were from severely food insecure households. The proportion of stunted children increased with food insecurity. There was a 7 and 12 percentage point increase in stunting between the food secure and either moderate and severely food insecure households respectively. In terms of wealth index, most of the households were ranked poorest at entry time in relation to the overall population in the two study sites. Stunting was highest (53 %) among poorest households and lowest (47 %) among the least poor households.

Mother's education and parity were significantly associated with stunting. Overall, three quarters of the mothers had at least primary level education. The proportion of children who were stunted was higher (52 %) among mothers with lower levels of education (primary or less) compared with at least secondary education (43 %). Stunting was more common among mothers with a parity of five or more (54 %) compared with those with a parity of below five.

3.3.1   Food Security, Wealth Status and Stunting

Table 2 shows levels of stunting stratified by both household food security and asset wealth status. The results show disproportionate stunting of children across wealth index. The proportion of stunted children was higher among the poorest households than among the least poor. In addition, within each wealth tertile, stunting was higher among children from food insecure households than those from food secure. Stunting was highest among severely food insecure households ranked in the poorest tertile and lowest among food secure households in the middle wealth tertile. These results illustrate the interactive effect of household food security and wealth status on child nutrition.

TABLE 3.2   Proportion of stunted children by food security status and asset wealth index at the point of stunting

	Number	% of sample	% stunted	P-Value
Poorest - overall	2815	41.0	52.50	0.26
Food secure	469	20.2	49.5	
Moderate	1572	94.9	52.5	
Food insecure	774	26.9	54.3	
Middle poor - overall	2072	30.2	46.04	0.01
Food secure	554	23.9	40.8	
Moderate	1009	60.9	46.6	
Food insecure	509	17.7	50.7	
Least poor - overall	1971	28.7	46.52	0.08
Food secure	926	39.9	44.3	
Moderate	859	51.8	47.6	
Food insecure	186	6.5	52.7	

Figure 1 shows the survival curves for both food security and asset wealth index. Children from the poorest and food insecure households had a lower survival time. By 23 months close to half of the children from poor and severely food insecure households were stunted. The food security survival pattern is consistent with descriptive statistics presented in Tables 1 and 2. The wealth index showed no clear difference between the middle poor and the least poor. However, the poorest, had a lower survival than the middle and least poor.

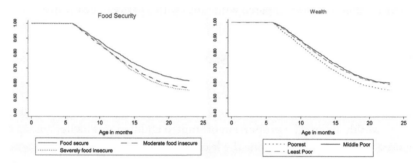

FIGURE 3.1   Food security and wealth status Kaplan Meir survival curves

Figure 2 shows the levels of stunting by age of the child in months. Stunting was highest between 10 and 15 months, peaking at around 12 months of age. That is, from 6 months, age at which complimentary feeding is introduced, there was a sharp increase in the proportion of stunted children until 15th month and thereafter declines to slightly about 10 % by month 23.

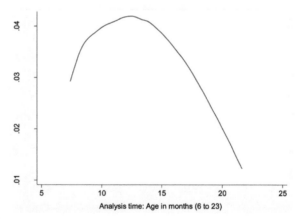

FIGURE 3.2   Cox regression survival curve on hazards of stunting.

Using Cox regression models, we further explored the relationship between household food security and stunting (Table 3). Three models are presented: Model 1, with bivariate associations for food security, wealth status, study site and gender of the child; Model 2 includes both food security and wealth index; and a full model (Model 3) which includes Model 2 and controls for other known determinants of stunting. From the bivariate results (Model 1), household security and asset wealth index were significantly associated with stunting. That is, the hazards of a child being stunted if he or she was from a moderate and severely food insecure household increased by 16 % and 23 % compared with children from food secure household. Improved household asset wealth index was associated with lower risk of being stunted. Children from middle (HR: 0.86, CI: 0.79–0.93) and least poor (HR: 0.89, CI: 0.82–0.96) households had significantly lower risk of being stunted compared to those from the poorest households.

After adjusting for the wealth index (M2), the association between food security and stunting remained positive and significant. In this model, children from the severely food insecure households were 21 % (HR: 1.21, CI: 1.09–1.33) more likely to be stunted than those from food secure households. The risk of stunting among moderately food insecure households significantly increased by 15 %; while the effect of wealth index on stunting was attenuated and was only significant for those in the middle category. That is, though the middle poor and least poor had a reduced risk of stunting, only the risk among middle poor remained significant at 95 % level of significance. The third model (M3) included both food security and wealth status controlling for a number of characteristics. Food security in this model remained significant, and was in the same directions as model 1 and 2, while the association between stunting and wealth status was stronger and significant for the middle and least poor category. Other factors significantly associated with stunting in model three were breast-feeding and gender of the child. That is, children who had been introduced to complimentary foods and girls were 37 and 20 % less likely to be stunted compared to those who were breastfeeding and boys respectively.

We hypothesized that household food security interacts with asset wealth index to influence stunting. That is, wealth index modifies the effect of food security on stunting. To assess this interaction, we fitted a full model (similar to Model 3) while interacting food security and wealth status (Fig. 3). In the model, we alternated the reference category to food secure households in each wealth status. That is, in the poorest wealth category, the reference group was those households in this category that were food secure, likewise in the least

TABLE 3.3 Bivariate and multiple Cox regression hazard ratio on stunting (n = 6858)

Variable	M1: Bivariate			M2: Adjusted for WI			M3: Other covariates		
	HR	95 % CI		HR	95 % CI		HR	95 % CI	
Food security									
Food secure	1			1			1		
Moderate	1.16**	1.07	1.26	1.15**	1.05	1.25	1.12**	1.02	1.22
Food insecure	1.23**	1.11	1.35	1.21**	1.09	1.33	1.15*	1.03	1.28
Wealth index									
Poorest				1			1		
Middle	0.86**	0.79	0.93	0.87**	0.80	0.94	0.82**	1.02	1.22
Least poor	0.89**	0.82	0.96	0.93	0.86	1.02	0.79*	1.03	1.28
Study site									
Korogocho	1						1		
Viwandani	0.85**	0.79	0.91				0.95	0.86	1.04
Child sex									
Male	1						1		
Female	0.80**	0.75	0.85				0.80**	0.75	0.86

WI = Wealth index; Model 1 (M1): Bivariate association; Model 2 (M2): Includes both food security and asset wealth index; Model 3 (M3): Includes model 2 and controls for other covariates: Mother and child characteristics (Age at birth, education level, parity at birth, breastfeeding, birth weight) and Household characteristics (head education, sex, age and size)

Significant at *p < 0.05; **p < 0.01

poor wealth category, the reference group was those households in this category that were food secure. In this regard, the same model was run three times with the reference category changing for each wealth category. By so doing, one is able to interpret the hazards ratios within each wealth category more objectively.

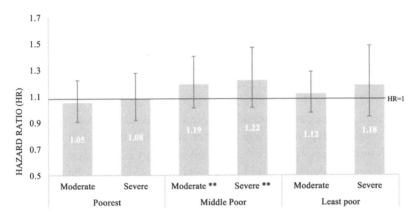

*P<0.05; **P<0.01　　FOOD SECURITY AND WEALTH STATUS INTERACTION

FIGURE 3.3　Interacting effect of household food security and wealth index on child stunting

Overall, within each wealth category, the risk for stunting increased with increasing food insecurity. However, the association was only significant among the middle poor households. Among the poorest households, the effect of food security on stunting was minimal and not statistically significant. Similarly among the least poor, children from households that were moderate or severely food insecure were 12 and 18 % more likely to be stunted, however, this difference was not statistically significant. Among the middle poor households, moderately and severely food insecure households were at significantly higher risk of being stunted compared with food secure ones.

3.4　DISCUSSION

We sought to determine the relationship between household food security and nutritional outcome of children aged between 6 and 23 months living in two informal settlements in Nairobi using a longitudinal dataset. We hypothesized that food insecurity was a key determinant of stunting and that the effect would be modified by household wealth status. The prevalence of stunting in the study sample was high at 49 % and varied by household food security and wealth status. The prevalence of stunting in this study population was higher compared to the national average of 35 % [33].

The effect of food insecurity after controlling for household wealth status and other known determinants of stunting, showed that children from moderately and severely food insecure households were more likely to be stunted than those from food secure households. Models of food security and child nutrition assume that food insecurity results in a lower intake of energy rich foods and nutrients resulting in changes to child health. A recent study by Ali Naser et al. [34] in Malaysia, showed that food insecurity was associated with stunting and underweight. In contrast, in high income countries the reverse is often true. In high income settings, children from food insecure households have an increased risk of being either overweight or obese than those from rich households presumable due to high consumption of energy rich foods coupled with inadequate physical activity and high stress levels [35]. Closer home, a study among orphaned children aged between 6 and 14 years and living in informal settlements of Nairobi, showed that food security was not associated with their nutritional status [36].

While urban populations are often thought to have better social indicators than rural areas, the growth of slums has eroded this advantage [11]. Research evidence has shown that the urban poor are often worse off than their rural counterparts [37, 38]. Recent research shows that urban poor households are becoming increasingly food insecure, and in Nairobi, levels of food insecurity are estimated to be as high as 85 % [39]. In the slum setting, food insecurity leads to either decreased food intake, or skipping of meals as well as a lack of nutritious foods to meet the dietary needs of household members. The latter is an important composite for growth especially among children. Studies conducted in the two slums have shown that dietary diversification is rare and that many households consume the same foods for most meals [39]. The positive relationship between food security and child nutrition therefore suggests that poor households are not able to meet their daily dietary needs.

When the results were stratified by wealth tertile (poorest, middle poor and least poor), we observed an increased risk of stunting with increasing food insecurity status. However the differences in stunting by food security status were only significant for the middle poor households. The positive effect of the interaction between food security and wealth status is of interest. While many studies have not explored this relationship, the few that have found a diminished effect of food security controlling for wealth index. For instance, a study in Ghana found that controlling for other covariates minus the wealth status food insecurity to be highly associated with stunting of children aged between 24 and 36 months and not those below 24 months [40]. However, when household wealth status (measured in terms of house quality and asset ownership) was controlled for, the effect became insignificant [40]. Hannum et al. [41] in their study on the effect of poverty, food security and nutritional deprivation on literacy achievement found food insecurity to be positively associated with wealth, with the poorest children likely to be both stunted and underweight. In Brazil, Reis [42] investigated food insecurity and its relationship with income and child health and concluded that food security to be a key in influencing the relationship between income and stunting among poor children.

Food security, poverty and nutritional status are closely intertwined, however, their mechanism of transmission remains unclear [40]. While food insecurity leads to decreased dietary intake, poverty is closely linked with increased levels of food insecurity [13]. Poverty, in this regard, modifies the effect of food insecurity on nutrition. In this study, the effect of food insecurity on stunting was only significant among the middle poor households. We think that this significant result is due to the unstable situation of the middle poor category, who are likely to be in a transition phase and can either fall back to the poorest category or move to the least poor. In this regard, households in the middle wealth status may be more diverse. Moreover, with very limited urban agriculture, households in the study setting depend on out-of-pocket food purchases. In this regard, the poverty status may therefore define the household's access to food. Research evidence on wealth status and obesity shows that in high income countries people from poorer households are more likely to be obese/overweight compared with those from richer households [43]. In high income countries, food insecurity is a measure of poverty, and a strong predictor of overweight, especially among women [44]. In contrast, in low and middle income settings, the poor are less likely to be obese or overweight [43]. Lower levels of obesity and overweight in poorer households in low and middle income countries is often attributed to lower access to energy rich foods and a more physically active lifestyle because the poor have to rely on walking and are more likely to have manual jobs. In the study context, the poorest households irrespective of their food security status, may lack the resources to get enough food for diverse dietary requirements and while the least poor, may have some resources that despite their different food security status guarantees some stability of food. This may be a possible explanation for the lack of statistical significance between the food security categories for the poorest and least poor households.

We interpret the results of this study in light of the following limitations: First, the effect of poverty and food security on nutrition may be more pronounced in older ages than among children. For instance, adult members of the households may miss meals to cope with the existing situations in order to ensure that their children have some food. Saaka et al. [40] found that the relationship between food security and nutritional status was stronger among children aged between 24 and 36 months than those aged between 6 and 23 months. However, the importance of studying those aged between 6 and 23 months is twofold: it is a critical age for growth and in the study context, nearly half of the children are stunted by this age. Secondly, household wealth was assessed using proxy measures—household amenities and asset ownership—due to a lack of accurate information on household incomes and expenditures, which may be better measures of household wealth. Despite these limitations, we utilize longitudinal data from the same children and households providing an opportunity for survival analysis, which is superior to cross-sectional analysis. The longitudinal nature of the data also allowed controlling for fluctuations in household food security and wealth status over time, by modelling the two variables as time variant. By so doing, the probability of reporting a significant effect when there is none was reduced [45].

3.5 CONCLUSION

The findings of this study show food insecurity is intertwined with malnutrition and poverty. Food insecurity is a public health problem and increasingly becoming a social determinant of health [46, 47]. Given that food security is a human right [47], there is need for social protection policies to reduce the high rates of child malnutrition in the urban informal settlements. Previous efforts by Concern Worldwide in Korogocho slums showed that social protection strategies through cash transfers increased the mean number of meals from 1.6 to 2.5 in a day and decreased prevalence of food insecurity from as high as 97 to 74 % [48]. Further, targeted efforts to address malnutrition among children are imperative. The interventions must take into account high levels of poor sanitation and diarrhoea, which may erode the gains of improved food security among the slums residents [49]. As such, interventions must take a holistic approach in addressing the high levels of malnutrition among the vulnerable urban poor households.

REFERENCES

1. FAO, WFP, IFAD. The state of food insecurity in the World 2012. In: Economic growth is necessary but not sufficient to accelerate reduction of hunger and malnutrition. Rome: FAO; 2012.

2. Cook JT, Frank DA. Food security, poverty, and human development in the United States. Ann N Y Acad Sci. 2008;1136(1):193–209. doi:10.1196/annals.1425.001.

3. United Nations Department of Economic and Social Affairs. Sustainable development knowledge platform. 2015. https://sustainabledevelopment.un.org/?menu=1300. Accessed 13 October 2015.

4. Cook JT, Frank DA, Berkowitz C, Black MM, Casey PH, Cutts DB, et al. Food insecurity is associated with adverse health outcomes among human infants and toddlers. J Nutr. 2004;134(6):1432–8.

5. Grantham-McGregor S, Cheung YB, Cueto S, Glewwe P, Richter L, Strupp B, et al. Developmental potential in the first 5 years for children in developing countries. Lancet. 2007;369(9555):60–70. doi:10.1016/S0140-6736(07)60032-4.

6. Ahmed T, Mahfuz M, Ireen S, Shasmsir AM, Rahman S, Islam MM, et al. Nutrition of children and womein in Bangladesh: trends and directions for the future. J Popul Nutr. 2012;30(1):1–11.

7. Pinstrup-Andersen P, Babinard J. Globalisation and human nutrition: opportunities and risks for poor in developing countries. Afr J Food Nutr Sci. 2001;1:9–18.

8. United Nations Development Programme (UNDP). Africa human development report 2012: towards a food Secure future. Popul Dev Rev. 2013;39(1):172–3. doi:10.1111/j.1728-4457.2013.00584.x.

9. United Nations Children's Fund, World Health Organization, The World Bank. UNICEF-WHO-World Bank joint child malnutrition estimates. UNICEF, New York; WHO, Geneva; The World Bank, Washington, DC; 2012.

10. Kenya National Bureau of Statistics. Kenya demographic and health surveys, 2014: key indicators. Nairobi, Kenya: Kenya National Bureau of Statistics (KNBS)2015; 2015.

11. Fotso JC, Madise N, Baschieri A, Cleland J, Zulu E, Mutua MK, et al. Child growth in urban deprived settings: does household poverty status matter? At which stage of child development? Health Place. 2012;18(2):375–84. doi:10.1016/j.healthplace.2011.12.003.

12. Engle P, Menon P, Haddad L. Care and nutrition: concepts and measurement. World Dev. 1999;27(8):1309–37.

13. Black RE, Allen LH, Bhutta ZA, Caulfield LE, de Onis M, Ezzati M, et al. Maternal and child undernutrition: global and regional exposures and health consequences. Lancet. 2008;371(9608):243–60.

14. Casey PH, Simpson PM, Gossett JM, Bogle ML, Champagne CM, Connell C, et al. The association of child and household food Insecurity with childhood overweight status. Pediatrics. 2006;118(5):e1406–13. doi:10.1542/peds.2006-0097.

15. Martorell R. The nature of child malnutrition and its long-term implications. Food Nutr Bull. 1999;20(3):288–92.

16. Jyoti DF, Frangillo EA, Jones SJ. Food insecurity affects school children's academic performance, weight gain, and social skills. J Nutr. 2005;135:2831–9.

17. Prado E, Dewey K. Insight nutrition and brain development in early life, AT&T Technical Brief, vol. 4. 2012.

18. Thompson R, Nelson C. Developmental science and the media: early brain development. Am Psychol Assoc. 2001;56:5–15.
19. Alaimo K, Olson C, Frangillo EA, Briefel R. Food insufficiency, poverty, and health in U.S. pre-school and school-age children. Am J Public Health. 2001;91:781–6.
20. Vozoris NT, Tarasuk VS. Household food insufficiency is associated with poorer health. J Nutr. 2003;133(1):120–6.
21. Psaki S, Bhutta ZA, Ahmed T, Ahmed S, Bessong P, Islam M, et al. Household food access and child malnutrition: results from the eight-country MAL-ED study. Popul Health Metrics. 2012;10(1):24. doi:10.1186/1478-7954-10-24.
22. Dubois L, Farmer A, Girard M, Porcherie M. Family food insufficiency is related to over-weight among preschoolers'. Soc Sci Med. 2006;63:1503–16.
23. Dubois L, Damion F, Burnier D, Tatone-Tokuda F, Girard M, Gordon-Strachan G, et al. Household food insecurity and childhood overweight in Jamaica and Québec: a gender-based analysis. BMC Public Health. 2011;11:119.
24. Osei A, Pandey P, Spiro D, Nielson J, Shrestha R, Talukder Z, et al. Household food insecurity and nutritional status of children aged 6 to 23 months in Kailali district of Nepal. Food Nutr Bull. 2010;31:4.
25. Beguy D, Elung'ata P, Mberu B, Oduor C, Wamukoya M, Nganyi B, et al. HDSS profile: the Nairobi Urban Health and Demographic Surveillance System (NUHDSS). Int J Epidemiol. 2015. doi:10.1093/ije/dyu251.
26. Zere E, McIntyre D. Inequiteis in under-five child malnutrion in South Africa. Int J Equity Health. 2003;2:7.
27. UNICEF. The state of the world's children 1998. New York: Oxford University Press; 1998.
28. World Food Summit. Rome declaration on world food security. 1996. http://www.fao.org/docrep/003/w3613e/w3613e00.HTM . Accessed on 13 October 2013.
29. Radimer KL, Olson C, Campell CC. Development of indicators to access hunger. J Nutr. 1990;120(11):1544–8.
30. Faye O, Baschieri A, Falkingham J, Muindi K. Hunger and food insecurity in Nairobi's slums: an assessment using IRT models. J Urban Health. 2011;88 Suppl 2:S235–54.
31. Tavakol M, Dennick R. Making sence of Cronbach's alpha. Int J Med Educ. 2011;2:23–55. doi:10.5116/ijme.4dfb.8dfd.
32. Filmer D, Pritchett LH. Estimating wealth effects without expenditure data – or tears: an application to educational enrolments in states of India. Demography. 2001;38(1):115–32.
33. Kenya National Bureau of Statistics (KNBS), ICF Macro. Kenya demographic and health survey 2008–09. Calverton: KNBS and ICF Macro; 2010.
34. Ali Naser I, Jalil R, Wan Muda WM, Wan Nik WS, Mohd Shariff Z, Abdullah MR. Association between household food insecurity and nutritional outcomes among children in Northeastern of Peninsular Malaysia. Nutr Res Pract. 2014;8(3):304–11. doi:10.4162/nrp.2014.8.3.304.
35. Dammann K, Smith C. Food-related attitudes and behaviors at home, school, and restau-rants: perspectives from racially diverse, urban, low-income 9- to 13-year-old children in Minnesota. J Nutr Educ Behav. 2010;42(6):389–97.
36. Kimani-Murage EW, Holding PA, Fotso JC, Ezeh AC, Madise N, Kahurani EN, et al. Food security and nutritional outcomes among urban poor orphans in Nairobi, Kenya. J Urban Health. 2011;88 Suppl 2:282–97. doi:10.1007/s11524-010-9491-z.

37. Fotso JC. Urban–rural differentials in child malnutrition: trends and socioeconomic correlates in sub-Saharan Africa. Health Place. 2007;13:205–23. doi:10.1016/j.healthplace. 2006.01.004.

38. Fotso JC. Child health inequities in developing countries: differences across urban and rural areas. Int J Equity Health. 2006;5:9.

39. Kimani-Murage EW, Schofield L, Wekesah F, Mohamed S, Mberu B, Ettarh R, et al. Vulnerability to food insecurity in urban slums: experiences from Nairobi, Kenya. J Urban Health. 2014. doi:10.1007/s11524-014-9894-3.

40. Saaka M, Osman SM. Does household food insecurity affect the nutritional status of preschool children aged 6–36 Months? Int J Popul Res. 2013;2013:12. doi:10.1155/2013/304169.

41. Hannum E, Liu J, Frongillo EA. Poverty, food insecurity and nutritional deprivation in rural China: implications for children's literacy achievement. Int J Educ Dev. 2014;34:90–7. http://dx.doi.org/10.1016/j.ijedudev.2012.07.003.

42. Reis M. Food insecurity and the relationship between household income and children's health and nutrition in Brazil. Health Econ. 2012;21(4):405–27. doi:10.1002/hec.1722.

43. Dinsa GD, Goryakin Y, Fumagalli E, Suhrcke M. Obesity and socioeconomic status in developing countries: a systematic review. Obes Rev. 2012;13(11):1067–79. doi:10.1111/j.1467-789X.2012.01017.x.

44. Townsend MS, Peerson J, Love B, Achterberg C, Murphy SP. Food insecurity is positively related to overweight in women. J Nutr. 2001;131(6):1738–45.

45. Bellera CA, MacGrogan G, Debled M, Lara CT, Brouste V, Mathoulin-Pélissier S. Variables with time-varying effects and the Cox model: some statistical concepts illustrated with a prognostic factor study in breast cancer. BMC Med Res Methodol. 2010;10:20. doi:10. 1186/1471-2288-10-20.

46. McIntyre L. Food security: More than a determinant of health. Policy Options. 2003; 24(3):46–51.

47. Chilton M, Rose D. A rights-based approach to food insecurity in the United States. Am J Public Health. 2009;99(7):1203–11. doi:10.2105/AJPH.2007.130229.

48. MacAuslan I, Schofield L. Evaluation of Concern Kenya's Korogocho emergency and food security cash transfer initiative. Nairobi: Concern Worldwide and Oxford Policy Management; 2011.

49. African Population and Health Research Center (APHRC). Population and health dynamics in Nairobi's informal settlements: report of the Nairobi cross-sectional slums survey (NCSS) 2012. Nairobi: APHRC; 2014.

CHAPTER 4

Household Food Access and Child Malnutrition: Results from the Eight-Country MAL-ED Study

Stephanie Psaki, Zulfiqar A. Bhutta,
Tahmeed Ahmed, Shamsir Ahmed,
Pascal Bessong, Munirul Islam, Sushil John,
Margaret Kosek, Aldo Lima, Cebisa Nesamvuni,
Prakash Shrestha, Erling Svensen, Monica Mcgrath,
Stephanie Richard, Jessica Seidman,
Laura Caulfield, Mark Miller, and
William Checkley

4.1 BACKGROUND

One in every five children in the developing world is malnourished, and poor nutrition is associated with half of all child deaths worldwide [1, 2]. Malnutrition in early childhood can lead to cognitive and physical deficits, and may cause similar deficits in future generations as malnourished mothers give birth to low birth weight infants [3]. Malnutrition also increases susceptibility and incidence of infections and is associated with diminished response to vaccines [4]. The root of malnutrition in early childhood is complex with a variety of direct and underlying contributors related to lack of food, including insufficient breast-feeding and inadequate complementary foods; protein and nutrient loss from respiratory and gastrointestinal infections; chronic immune stimulation due to persistent parasitic intestinal infections; and inadequate water and sanitation [5, 6]. Food insecurity is a key risk factor for child malnutrition [7, 8]. Based on the 1996 World Food Summit, food security occurs "when all people at all times have access to sufficient, safe, nutritious food to maintain a healthy and active life" [9]. Food security comprises three hierarchical components: availability, access and utilization [10]. Availability is often measured through proxies at the population level, such as national agricultural output, while access and utilization are more often measured at the household and individual levels respectively [11]. While direct measures of food utilization exist, such as food frequency questionnaires [12], household food access has often been measured indirectly, through child anthropometry [10] or agricultural productivity [12]. Measurement of all three aspects of food insecurity has posed persistent challenges, such as the difficulty in measuring the impact of short-term shocks on household food access [12]. Recent research, however, shows promise in the area of food access measurement, with the construction of simple household survey measures such as the Household Food Insecurity Access Scale (HFIAS) [11, 13, 14]. Low-cost and valid measures of household food insecurity are necessary to accurately predict the prevalence of food insecurity in response to changing conditions [15]. Such measurements can then inform targeted interventions to diminish childhood morbidity and mortality [10, 12]. However, global progress against food insecurity requires measures that are valid and comparable across countries. We sought to assess the acceptability, validity, and generalizability of the HFIAS, an existing nine-item measure of household food access, in the setting of a multi-country study. To achieve this aim, we collected cross-sectional data on household food access insecurity and child nutritional status, as measured by anthropometry, in eight country sites to determine whether these variables were related, and whether this relationship was consistent across diverse populations.

4.2 MATERIALS AND METHODS

4.2.1 Study Setting

We conducted our study at the eight field sites in the Malnutrition and Enteric Infections: Consequences for Child Health and Development (MAL-ED) Network cohort study. The MAL-ED Network, comprising researchers from thirteen academic and research institutions, aims to explore the relationship between malnutrition and intestinal infections and their consequences for various aspects of child growth and development. Sites are utilizing a standardized protocol for the collection of twice-weekly diarrhea surveillance information, monthly anthropometry, urine for gut function and iodine status, stool for enteric pathogens, blood for micronutrients and vaccine response, and cognitive development assessments. Study sites are located in rural, urban, and peri-urban areas of Bangladesh, Brazil, India, Nepal, Pakistan, Peru, South Africa and Tanzania (See Additional file 1). The MAL-ED study began enrolling pregnant women in 2009, and plans to follow a cohort of approximately 200 newborns per site for up to 36 months. We report on pilot study activities that preceded enrollment for the cohort study, aimed at characterizing the relationship between food access and child nutritional status.

4.2.2   Study Design

In preparation for the MAL-ED cohort study, we sought to develop and test cross-country indicators of food access insecurity and socioeconomic status (SES). We administered a standardized survey including demographic, SES, and food access questions to 100 households in each of the eight field sites between September 2009 and August 2010. Households were randomly selected from census results collected within the previous year at each study site. Households were eligible to participate if they were located within the MAL-ED study area and had an index child aged 24 to 60 months. Data collection lasted approximately two to four weeks in each site. We obtained ethical approval from the Institutional Review Boards at each of the participating research sites, at the Johns Hopkins Bloomberg School of Public Health (Baltimore, USA) and at the University of Virginia School of Medicine (Charlottesville, USA). Demographic and SES questions were adapted from the most recent Demographic and Health Surveys [16] in collaboration with site investigators. Questions focused on age and education of the head of household and child's mother, as well as the mother's fertility history. The SES section included a series of questions on household assets, housing materials, and water and sanitation facilities. The questionnaire was developed in English, and then translated into local languages by site investigators using appropriate local terms (See Additional file 2). The questionnaire was accompanied by standard operating procedures based on existing guidelines for administration of the HFIAS [17]. Field supervisors trained field workers prior to survey administration, and used locally appropriate management techniques to support complete, accurate and timely data collection, including weekly review of all data to ensure quality.

4.2.3   Food Access Insecurity Score

To assess food access insecurity, our survey included the nine-question HFIAS (See Online Supplement), adapted in 2006 by the Food And Nutrition Technical Assistance (FANTA) project for use in low resource settings [18]. Although this scale has been validated and adapted in individual country settings through previous studies [18–20], to our knowledge it has not been used in its original form in a multi-country study. The nine-item scale uses a four-week recall period and captures three dimensions of the access component of household food insecurity: anxiety and uncertainty about household food access (item 1); insufficient quality (items 2–4); and insufficient food intake and its physical consequences (items 5–9) [18]. Responses on the nine items were summed to create the food access insecurity score, with a minimum score of 0 indicating the most food access secure households, and a maximum score of 27 indicating the most food access insecure households. We also categorized households into four groups [17]: food access secure, and mildly, moderately and severely food access insecure.

4.2.4   Anthropometry

We measured height and weight in one child aged 24 to 60 months in each participating household. When multiple children in this age range lived in one household, we randomly chose one child to avoid intra-household correlation in our data. Trained field staff measured standing height to the nearest 0.1 cm using a locally produced platform with sliding headboard. Digital scales were used to measure weight to the nearest 100 grams. Height-for-age (HAZ) and weight-for-height (WHZ) Z-scores were calculated based on World Health Organization child growth standards [21]. We defined stunting and wasting as a HAZ and WHZ that were two standard deviations below the WHO standard, respectively.

4.2.5   Biostatistical Methods

Exploratory analyses involved examination of the distribution of each variable and inter-relationships between variables within and across sites. We then conducted a series of pooled analyses, including data from all eight country sites. We used a generalized additive model with a smoothing spline to characterize the relationship between food access insecurity and nutritional indicators. Our findings indicated that the pooled relationship between food access insecurity and both nutritional indicators was approximately linear, indicating the appropriateness of linear regression models. We then examined bivariate relationships between food access insecurity, HAZ, WHZ and SES indicators. Last, we used linear regression to model the relationship between food access insecurity and each nutritional outcome in the pooled sample of households, adjusted for child age, sex, maternal education, household bank account, people per room in the household, and access to an improved water source and sanitation facilities. We selected these SES indicators based on their relevance to the outcomes and sufficient variation within each country site. We compared the results to a model including a household SES score generated through principal components analysis based on 17 indicators of household wealth. The results were similar, and we felt that the selection of individual indicators provided more interpretable information on the relationships between food access insecurity and SES. To control for differences in baseline levels of HAZ and WHZ, we included indicator variables for all but one country. We conducted a likelihood ratio test comparing a full model with interactions between food access insecurity score and the eight country dummy variables with a reduced model lacking those interactions. The results of this test provided evidence of the extent of heterogeneity in the relationship between food access insecurity and HAZ across countries. We used R (http://www.r-project.org) and STATA 12 (STATA Corp., College Station, USA) for statistical analysis.

4.3   RESULTS

4.3.1   Characteristics of Study Populations

We surveyed a total of 800 households. One child had missing anthropometry and ten had extreme anthropometric values (greater than six standard deviations from the mean) based on the WHO standard [21]. This resulted in a final sample size of 789 households (98.6% of original sample). The mean age of sampled children was 41 months (SD = 10.4); 51.5% of children were male, ranging from 58.6% in Tanzania to 44.3% in Pakistan. Variation in household SES across country sites was evidenced by variations in maternal education (3.3 years in Pakistan to 10.1 years in South Africa) and proportion with a bank account (2% in India to 76% in South Africa) (Table 1). Furthermore, the mean household SES score, calculated through principal components analysis, ranged from a low

TABLE 4.1 Selected household characteristics overall and by country (n = 789)

		Overall	Bangladesh	Brazil	India	Nepal	Pakistan	Peru	South Africa	Tanzania
	Sample size	789	99	98	100	100	98	99	96	99
SES Indicators	Owns bank account (%)	31	23	21	10	62	39	15	76	2
	People per room (mean)*	1.7	3.7	1.3	3.9	2.5	5.5	1.6	1.2	1.7
	Mean maternal education (years)	6.4	3.7	7.8	6.7	6.6	3.3	7.8	10.1	5.3
	Owns Mattress (%)	58	66	98	1	99	13	82	66	39
	Owns mobile phone (%)	68	63	81	53	96	68	31	96	54
	Owns radio or transistor (%)	41	11	74	2	48	12	55	82	46
	Has electricity (%)	84	100	99	97	99	98	85	94	0
	Owns table (%)	57	29	86	21	65	50	100	74	33
Hygiene Indicators	Improved water source (%)	86	100	100	100	98	100	98	65	28
	Improved sanitation facility (%)	72	100	100	37	100	74	84	84	1
Food Access Insecurity Categories§	Food secure (%)	37.5	33.3	32.7	30.0	73.0	22.5	20.2	20.8	66.7
	Mildly insecure (%)	11.4	15.2	9.2	5.0	7.0	12.2	27.3	9.4	6.1
	Moderately insecure (%)	27.5	33.3	11.2	29.0	12.0	48.0	29.3	40.6	17.2
	Severely insecure (%)	23.6	18.2	46.9	36.0	8.0	17.4	23.2	29.2	10.1

*People per room is the number of people who usually sleep in the house divided by the number of rooms in the house that are used for sleeping.

§Food access insecurity categories are based on the guidelines in Coates et al. 2007.

of −2.30 in Tanzania to high of 2.08 and 2.16 in Brazil and South Africa, respectively (See Additional file 1). Nearly all households, with the exception of those in Tanzania, had access to electricity and reported access to improved water and sanitation, as defined by the World Health Organization [22].

4.3.2   Household Food Access Insecurity Scores

Food access insecurity score distributions were skewed right, indicating a large subgroup of households reporting no food access insecure experiences in the preceding four weeks (Figure 1). Across sites, 37% of all households reported no food access insecurity in the last four weeks (score of 0). This value ranged from 18% of households in Peru to 72% in Nepal. Nepal (2.4) and Tanzania (2.6) had the lowest mean scores, as well as the smallest variability between households (SD = 4.8 for both), while Pakistan (8.3) and Brazil (7.9) had the highest mean scores. Nearly half (46.9%) of households in the Brazilian site reported severe food access insecurity, whereas the majority of households in Nepal (73.0%) and Tanzania (66.7%) indicated food access security.

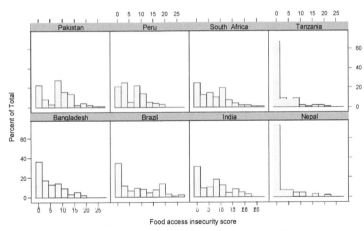

FIGURE 4.1   Barplots of food access insecurity score by country; 2009–10

4.3.3   Nutritional Indicators

Overall, 42% (ranging from 8% to 55%) of children were stunted, and 6% (range from 0% to 17%) were wasted (Figures 2 and 3). HAZ in India and Brazil were shifted toward the highest values, with approximately 35% of Brazilian children and 30% of Indian children measuring above the WHO standard mean. In the remaining six sites, approximately 50% of each population was stunted, and in Bangladesh all children were below the WHO standard mean in height. On average, a much smaller proportion of children in these sites experienced growth faltering as assessed by WHZ. In both South Africa and Tanzania, where over 50% of the sample children were stunted, none of them were wasted. In contrast, in India, where about 22% of children were stunted (fewer than most sites), a similar proportion (17%) were wasted (more than most sites). Stunting was significantly associated with infant age, water source, sanitation facility, mother's education, and people per room. Wasting was associated with water source and people per room. Low food access security was significantly associated with sex of the child, mother's education, ownership of a bank account, and people per room. Wasting and stunting were only weakly correlated with each other ($r = -0.02$; $p < 0.001$), but stunting was directly associated with inadequate water and sanitation facilities (Table 2). To further explore these relationships, we controlled for the same set of SES indicators in our regression models (Table 3). The final models for the relationship between food access insecurity and child malnutrition (HAZ and WHZ) retained the SES indicators that remained statistically significant, i.e. water source, mother's education, and people per room. This model was more parsimonious, and the relationship of interest remained consistent between models.

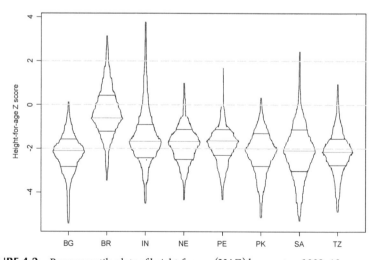

FIGURE 4.2   Box-percentile plots of height-for-age (HAZ) by country; 2009–10.

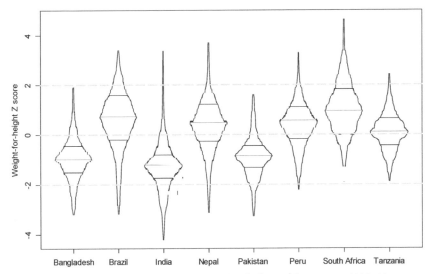

FIGURE 4.3   Box-percentile plots of weight-for-height (WHZ) by country; 2009–10.

Association between food access insecurity and nutritional indicators

In exploratory analyses, the relationship between food access insecurity and HAZ was approximately linear (Figure 4). Food access insecurity score was statistically significantly associated with HAZ (p = 0.008), but not with WHZ (Table 3). In pooled regression analyses, a 10-point increase in food access insecurity score was associated with a 0.20 SD decrease in HAZ score (95% CI 0.05 to 0.34), controlling for water source, maternal education and people per room. Sensitivity analyses indicated that the use of individual indicators of SES and the use of a linear combination of indicators using principal components analysis produce similar results with respect to our research question (results not presented). We chose to include individual SES indicators in our model for ease of interpretation. A likelihood ratio test comparing nested models with and without interactions terms indicated that the relationship between food access insecurity score and HAZ did not vary significantly across countries (p = 0.17). Moreover, none of the individual interaction terms between food insecurity and site achieved statistical significance at the 0.05 level (See Additional file 1 and Additional file 2).

TABLE 4.2 Relationship between socioeconomic status and nutritional indicators

	N	% Stunted (HAZ < −2)	p-value[+]	% Wasted (WHZ < −2)	p-value[+]	% Severely food access insecure[§]	p-value[+]
Sex							
Male	406	42.1	0.95	6.7	0.50	19.5	0.005
Female	382	41.9		5.5		19.3	
Age							
24-35 months	284	41.2	0.01	5.3	0.07	28.0	0.06
36-47 months	243	49.0		4.1		23.9	
48-60 months	262	36.3		8.8		27.9	
Water Source							
Not improved	109	58.7	<0.001	0.0	<0.01	24.8	0.75
Improved	680	39.3		23.4		23.4	
Sanitation Facility							
Not improved	218	49.5	<0.01	6.4	0.81	25.7	0.39
Improved	571	39.1		22.8		22.8	
Maternal education							
None	135	57.0	<0.001	5.2	0.15	22.2	0.59
1-5 years	174	43.1		26.4		26.4	
>5 years	480	37.3		22.9		22.9	
Bank Account							
No	545	42.2	0.83	6.6	0.36	28.3	<0.0001
Yes	244	41.4		13.1		13.1	
People per room							
<2	433	35.3	<0.001	10.1	<0.001	20.0	0.023
≥2	356	50.0		26.9		26.9	

§Severe food access insecurity is defined based on the guidance in Coates et al. 2007.
†p-values reflect results of t-tests and one-way ANOVA tests.

TABLE 4.3 Final models exploring the relationship between food access insecurity score and two measures of growth faltering, controlling for indicators of SES

	Height-for-age		Weight-for-height	
	Full model	**Final model**	**Full model**	**Final model**
Intercept (Tanzania as reference)	-1.96 (<0.001)	-2.20 (<0.001)	0.71 (0.003)	0.51 (0.007)
Bangladesh	-0.09 (0.73)	-0.14 (0.53)	-1.02 (<0.001)	-1.04 (<0.001)
Brazil	1.57 (<0.001)	1.52 (<0.001)	0.56 (0.02)	0.55 (<0.001)
Peru	0.16 (0.50)	0.14 (0.51)	0.30 (0.19)	0.27 (0.09)
India	0.50 (0.03)	0.48 (0.03)	-1.26 (<0.001)	-1.37 (<0.001)
Pakistan	0.18 (0.48)	0.14 (0.56)	-0.97 (<0.001)	-1.07 (<0.001)
Nepal	0.18 (0.47)	0.12 (0.55)	0.33 (0.17)	0.28 (0.06)
South Africa	-0.10 (0.68)	-0.16 (0.40)	0.88 (<0.001)	0.85 (<0.001)
Food access insecurity score (effect per unit score)	-0.020 (0.009)	-0.020 (0.008)	0.011 (0.13)	0.010 (0.13)
Age	-0.005 (0.24)		-0.01 (0.005)	-0.01 (0.004)
Sex	-0.03 (0.71)		-0.08 (0.30)	
Water Source[‡]	0.38 (0.03)	0.37 (0.03)	-0.16 (0.33)	
Sanitation Facility[‡]	-0.03 (0.81)		0.12 (0.35)	
Maternal education (years)	0.02 (0.06)	0.02 (0.06)	-0.005 (0.69)	
Bank account	-0.06 (0.57)		-0.05 (0.62)	
People per room	-0.06 (0.03)	-0.06 (0.03)	-0.02 (0.53)	
Adjusted R^2	20.3%	20.6%	35.1%	35.2%

Rows contain effect estimates and p-values in parentheses.

[‡]Dichotomous variables measuring access to improved facilities based on WHO standards.

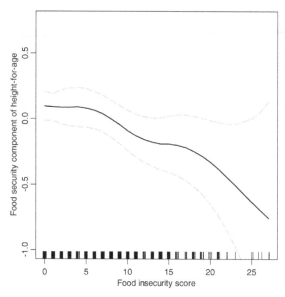

FIGURE 4.4 Relationship between food access insecurity score and height-for-age (HAZ); 2009–10. We fitted a smoothing spline to study the relationship between food access insecurity score and HAZ using a generalized additive model. The figure shows the fitted smoothing spline and corresponding 95% confidence intervals.

DISCUSSION

In this study, we found that food access insecurity was associated with a statistically significant shift in the distribution of children's HAZ toward lower values, after adjusting for sociodemographic factors. Although prevalence of both food access insecurity and faltering in HAZ varied across countries, a likelihood ratio test for heterogeneity revealed that the relationship between these variables was consistent across countries. Our findings on the epidemiology of growth faltering are consistent with the literature. Previous studies have reported higher prevalence of stunting than wasting within populations [23–25], and more variation in wasting than in stunting across populations [1, 25]. Although our results indicate regional patterns in prevalence of wasting only, others have found clear regional patterns in both stunting and wasting [1, 23, 25]. Variations between sites likely reflect the impact of numerous factors, including seasonal effects on the food supply, patterns of enteric infections, genetic predispositions, and access to prenatal and infant health services. Stunting and wasting are indicators of chronic and acute malnutrition, respectively [11]. However, beyond reflecting differences in the length of exposure to deprivation, they are also differentially associated with other socio-demographic variables, such as maternal education and immunizations [23, 25]. Given different risk factors for wasting and stunting, and the weak correlation between these measures in our data, it is not surprising that food access insecurity was associated with faltering in HAZ but not WHZ. In addition to different risk factors, growth faltering in WHZ tends to occur at younger ages and result in higher mortality than faltering in HAZ [1]. Given the age of children enrolled in this study (older than 24 months), they were more likely to be stunted or healthy than to be wasted. Further research is warranted on approaches to expanding this household food access insecurity measure to more effectively capture factors associated with wasting. Patterns in SES, food access insecurity, and growth faltering were not clearly clustered by region, and no country ranked consistently highest or lowest in all factors. For example, Tanzanian households were among the poorest when measured by socioeconomic indicators, but were also among the most food access secure. We hypothesize that this difference in rankings by food access insecurity and household SES might be due to the predominantly agricultural setting, where reporting bias on food access insecurity might be more common, and where wealth may not be as closely tied to food access security as in urban settings. The opposite pattern was true of Brazilian households, which also had among the highest mean values of HAZ and WHZ scores. Our results indicate that food access insecurity was not simply an indicator of SES, but was also independently associated with growth faltering. The effect of a five-point decrease in food access insecurity was roughly comparable to the effect of a five-year increase in mother's education on HAZ, and was approximately equal to one-third the effect of access to an improved water source. Although our analyses reveal that food access insecurity is independent of these socio-demographic indicators, these relationships warrant further exploration. The complexity of these relationships underlines the utility of a simple measure, such as the HFIAS, that could potentially predict growth faltering in children. The Food And Nutrition Technical Assistance (FANTA) project has worked since 2000 to validate and adapt the HFIAS [18]. Recent validation work in multiple countries has produced mixed results, leading investigators to suggest a shortened version of the scale, called the Household Hunger Scale, comprising only the final three items related to hunger [26]. The adapted version of the scale did not achieve statistical significance, suggesting that the full scale may be a better measure of chronic malnutrition, or that these two scales capture different information. However, in the context of the MAL-ED study, the full scale is more appropriate than the reduced scale for two reasons. First, more items generally result in higher scale reliability [27]. Second, we seek to measure the full experience of food access insecurity to facilitate exploration of the relationships between food access, food utilization, enteric infections, and nutritional markers in the early years of life. These results also provide evidence of the acceptability and validity of the nine-item HFIAS in a multi-country research setting. We were able to use the questions in their original form (with translation) in diverse cultural settings with limited problems in administration and no missing data. Our results, demonstrating a statistically significant relationship between food access insecurity and HAZ—two variables that we would expect to be correlated—provide evidence of the construct validity of the HFIAS scale in a multi-country setting [28]. Furthermore, although this measure only focuses on the access aspect of food insecurity, previous research has indicated that it correlates with dietary quality and the intake of a micronutrient rich diet, two aspects of food utilization [20]. Finally, the lack of heterogeneity in this relationship across countries provides evidence of generalizability of its use in diverse low-income settings. The MAL-ED cohort study will allow us to look at food utilization and its relationship with food access more closely through inclusion of longitudinal measures of dietary intake and repeated measurement of food access insecurity. Our study has some potential limitations. The data are cross-sectional, preventing the collection of important longitudinal risk factors for malnutrition, such as intestinal infections. However, the statistically significant association between food access insecurity and HAZ indicates the utility of a short food security survey to screen for chronic malnutrition in settings where other data are not available. Our pilot study included children aged 24 to 60 months, although wasting effects are often greatest in the first two years of life [1]. The MAL-ED cohort study will follow children from birth, collecting data on diarrheal incidence and infectious agents, seasonal changes in food access insecurity, and other important exposures, such as dietary intake. In addition, some MAL-ED study sites raised concerns that responses to certain food access insecurity items might be culturally dependent, as has been shown by Coates and colleagues [14]. For example, although researchers in the Pakistan site felt that the HFIAS was robust to concerns, they noted the potential for bias given cultural stigma against reporting food insecurity. These differences are particularly relevant with regard to selecting universal cut points for food access insecurity, rather than associations between the continuous measure and outcomes. While further inquiry is warranted on cross-country variations in response thresholds, previous research indicates that the domains of food access insecurity that form the basis of the nine-item scale are similar across cultural settings (i.e. insufficient quantity, inadequate quality, and uncertainty or worry) [14]. Also, our pilot study was not designed to assess the important role of seasonality in household food access insecurity (Additional file 1 and Additional file 2); however, we are assessing seasonality in the MAL-ED cohort study, in which we are measuring food access insecurity every six months based on child enrollment. Finally, factors affecting child growth are present not only at the individual and household levels but also at the community, national, and regional levels. Information provided through a household survey can only explain a limited amount of variation in child growth outcomes [29]. In summary, a simple household food access insecurity score can help explain differences in HAZ distributions in a multi-country study, even after adjustment for demographic and SES indicators, and country-level differences. While we do not suggest that this tool should replace the collection of child anthropometry to assess nutritional status, it could be used as a rapid assessment tool to identify households at risk of child growth faltering. Given the simplicity of this measure, and its acceptability and validity in cross-country settings, we advocate its inclusion in research and programs seeking to understand and ameliorate the predictors of child malnutrition in developing countries.

REFERENCES

1. Black RE, Allen LH, Bhutta ZA, Caulfield LE, de Onis M, Ezzati M: Maternal and child undernutrition: global and regional exposures and health consequences. Lancet 2008,371(9608):243–260.
2. Caulfield LE, de Onis M, Blossner M, Black RE: Undernutrition as an underlying cause of child deaths associated with diarrhea, pneumonia, malaria, and measles. Am J Clin Nutr 2004,80(1):193–198.
3. Victora CG, Adair L, Fall C, Hallal PC, Martorell R, Richter L: Maternal and child undernutrition: consequences for adult health and human capital. Lancet 2008,371(9609):340–357.
4. Scrimshaw NS: Historical concepts of interactions, synergism and antagonism between nutrition and infection. J Nutr 2003, 133(1):316S-321S.
5. Campbell DI, Elia M, Lunn PG: Growth faltering in rural Gambian infants is associated with impaired small intestinal barrier function, leading to endotoxemia and systemic inflammation. J Nutr 2003,133(5):1332–1338.
6. Checkley W, Gilman RH, Black RE, Epstein LD, Cabrera L, Sterling CR: Effect of water and sanitation on childhood health in a poor Peruvian peri-urban community. Lancet 2004, 363(9403):112–118.
7. Cook JT: Clinical implications of household food security: definitions, monitoring, and policy. Nutr Clin Care 2002, 5(4):152–167.

8. Baig-Ansari N, Rahbar MH, Bhutta ZA, Badruddin SH: Child's gender and household food insecurity are associated with stunting among young Pakistani children residing in urban squatter settlements. Food Nutr Bull 2006, 27:114-27.

9. World Food Summit Plan of Action. Rome, Italy: FAO Corporate Document Repository; 1996:13-17. Available at: http://www.fao.org/DOCREP/003/W3613E/W3613E00. HTM

10. Sen AK: Poverty and famines: An essay on entitlement and deprivation. Clarendon Press; 1981.

11. Barrett CB: Measuring food insecurity. Science 2010,327(5967):825-828.

12. Carlsen MH, Lillegaard IT, Karlsen A, Blomhoff R, Drevon CA, Andersen LF: Evaluation of energy and dietary intake estimates from a food frequency questionnaire using independent energy expenditure measurement and weighed food records. Nutr J 2010, 9:37.

13. Webb P, Coates J, Frongillo EA, Rogers BL, Swindale A, Bilinsky P: Measuring household food insecurity: why it's so important and yet so difficult to do. J Nutr 2006,136(5):1404S-1408S.

14. Coates J, Frongillo EA, Rogers BL, Webb P, Wilde PE, Houser R: Commonalities in the experience of household food insecurity across cultures: what are measures missing? J Nutr 2006,136(5):1438S-1448S.

15. Hadley C, Maes K: A new global monitoring system for food insecurity? Lancet 2009,374(9697):1223-1224.

16. Demographic and Health Surveys, USAID. Information available at: http://www.measuredhs.com/

17. Coates J, Swindale A, Bilinsky P: Household Food Insecurity Access Scale for Measurement of Food Access: Indicator Guide. Version 3. Food and Nutrition Technical Assistance Program & USAID. 2007. Available at: http://www.fantaproject.org/publications/hfias_intro.shtml

18. Swindale A, Bilinsky P: Development of a universally applicable household food insecurity measurement tool: process, current status, and outstanding issues. J Nutr 2006,136(5):1449S-1452S.

19. Frongillo EA, Nanama S: Development and validation of an experience-based measure of household food insecurity within and across seasons in northern Burkina Faso. J Nutr 2006,136(5):1409S-1419S.

20. Melgar-Quinonez HR, Zubieta AC, MkNelly B, Nteziyaremye A, Gerardo MF, Dunford C: Household food insecurity and food expenditure in Bolivia, Burkina Faso, And the Philippines. J Nutr 2006,136(5):1431S-1437S.

21. World Health Organization: Child Growth Standards: Anthropometry Macros. 2011. Available at: http://www.who.int/childgrowth/software/en/index.html

22. World Health Organization Statistical Information System (WHOSIS): Indicator definitions and metadata. 2011. Available at: http://www.who.int/whosis/indicators/en/

23. Olusanya BO, Wirz SL, Renner JK: Prevalence, pattern and risk factors for undernutrition in early infancy using the WHO Multicentre Growth Reference: a community-based study. Paediatr Perinat Epidemiol 2010,24(6):572-583.

24. Singh MB, Fotedar R, Lakshminarayana J, Anand PK: Studies on the nutritional status of children aged 0-5 years in a drought-affected desert area of western Rajasthan, India. Public Health Nutr 2006,9(8):961-967.

25. Victora CG: The association between wasting and stunting: an international perspective. J Nutr 1992,122(5):1105-1110.

26. Deitchler M, Ballard T, Swindale A, Coates J: Validation of a Measure of Household Hunger for Cross-Cultural Use. 2010.
27. Carmines E, Zeller RA: Reliability and Validity Assessment. Sage: Beverly Hills, CA; 1979.
28. Cronbach LJ, Meehl PE: Construct validity in psychological tests. Psychol Bull 1955,52(4):281–302.
29. Frongillo EA Jr, de Onis M, Hanson KM: Socioeconomic and demographic factors are associated with worldwide patterns of stunting and wasting of children. J Nutr 1997,127(12):2302–2309.

Supplemental material is available online at http://pophealthmetrics.biomedcentral.com/ articles/10.1186/1478-7954-10-24.

CHAPTER 5

Food Insecurity and Linear Growth of Adolescents in Jimma Zone, Southwest Ethiopia

Tefera Belachew, David Lindstrom, Craig Hadley, Abebe Gebremariam, Wondwosen Kasahun, and Patrick Kolsteren

5.1 INTRODUCTION

Linear growth during adolescence is faster than in any other period of human growth after birth with the exception of the first year of life. As a transitional period between childhood and adulthood, adolescence provides an opportunity to prepare for a healthy productive and reproductive life. Puberty is a dynamic period of growth during adolescence characterized by rapid changes in body composition, shape and size, all of which are distinct for boys and girls. The onset of puberty approximately matches with a skeletal (biological) age of nearly 11 years in girls and 13 years in boys [1, 2]. On average, girls pass through each stage of puberty earlier than boys. The timing and duration of this pubertal development is influenced by a number of factors, including genetic characteristics, body composition, physical activity and diet [3–7]. Nutritional status and heavy exercise were identified to be the two major influences on the linear growth of adolescents [8]. However, in food insecure environments, it is hardly possible to fulfill the nutritional requirements of adolescents for healthy growth.

Food insecurity is prevalent among adolescents in Jimma, Ethiopia [9–11]. Evidence shows that food insecurity is associated with poor development and morbidity in children [12, 13], morbidity [9, 14, 15] and poor subsequent dietary habits [16] in adolescents. Food-insecure and stressed adolescents are likely to alter their dietary behavior in ways that increase the risk of stunting [16, 17]. It has been documented that even stunting that occurs soon after birth can have an impact on adolescent height [18] with a subsequent permanent negative effect on final height. However; growth spurts during adolescence can compensate for earlier stunted growth and provide an opportunity for catch-up growth before final height is attained.

Although childhood stunting is highly prevalent in Ethiopia in general and in the region where this study was conducted in particular [19], there is little research that investigated linear growth during adolescence. A cross-sectional study from Northern Ethiopia documented that 26.5% of adolescent girls were stunted [20]. However; this study did not have data on boys and did not examine the effect of food insecurity on growth. Although adolescents in Jimma zone suffer a number of negative health consequences of food insecurity (9, 15), the effect of food insecurity on linear growth has not been examined. To the best of our knowledge there was no study that examined the growth patterns of adolescents by food security status. This study aimed to determine the effect of food insecurity on the linear growth (height) of adolescents in southwest Ethiopia. We hypothesize that food insecure adolescents are likely to have lower growth (height) over two years follow up period compared to their food secure peers.

5.2   METHODS

5.2.1   Study Sample

Data for this study comes from the Jimma Longitudinal Family Survey of Youth (JLFSY) which followed a randomly selected sample of youth starting at ages 13–17 for approximately 5–6 years. The survey began in 2005 and sampled households and adolescents within households from six neighborhoods in Jimma Town (a zonal city of approximately 120,000 inhabitants), three nearby towns, and 18 rural "kebeles" (villages) immediately surrounding the towns. The study rural districts included a coffee growing area (altitude of 1911 meters), a highland vegetable growing area (altitude of 2300 meters), and a lower lying plain area dedicated to grains and other food crops (altitude of 1795 meters).

A street-by-street enumeration of all households was conducted to compile complete list. This generated a list of 5795 households which gave a sampling frame for random selection of 3,700 households. A two-stage sampling plan was used to select the target sample of adolescents. Households were classified into urban (Jimma City), semi-urban (Serbo, Dedo and Yebbu Towns) and six rural "kebeles" (two in the vicinity of each of the three small towns). At the first stage, households were randomly sampled with the sample size in each "kebele" determined by the relative proportion of the study population in the "kebele" and the overall target sample size. In the second stage, one adolescent (a boy or a girl) was randomly selected from each household using a Kish Table [21]. Using this sampling strategy, a total of 1059 boys and 1025 girls were interviewed in round one. The same adolescents were followed and interviewed at one year interval for the subsequent follow up surveys.

5.2.2   Measurements

Structured household and adolescent level questionnaires were used to collect data. The questionnaires were interviewer-administered and translated into Amharic and Oromifa languages and checked for consistency by other persons who speak both languages and English both at baseline, year 1 and year 2 of the survey. The household questionnaire included a household registry that collected socio-demographic information on all current resident and non-resident household members including information on their income and food security status. The heads of households responded to the household questionnaire. The adolescent questionnaire focused on issues related to adolescents' experiences of food insecurity, education, health and anthropometric measurements. The interview was conducted in a private place by an interviewer of the same sex as the adolescent respondent after the household interview was completed.

The interviewers received one week of intensive training prior to the pre-test and an additional week of training with the final version of the questionnaire before beginning the actual interviews. Supervisors kept track of the field procedures and checked the completed questionnaires every day to ensure accuracy of the data collected and the research team supervised the field team every week.

Adolescent food insecurity was measured using a four item index adopted from household food security questionnaires used in developing countries [22–24] by modifying the items that could be used at an individual adolescent level. The details of the methods are described elsewhere [9]. To summarize briefly, adolescents were asked whether in the last three months they (1) had ever worried about having enough food, (2) had to reduce food intake because of shortages of food or money to buy food, (3) had to go without having eaten because of shortage of food or money to buy food and (4) had to ask outside the home for food because of shortage of food or money to buy food. A "Yes" response to any of the food security questions was labeled to have score of "1" and "No" was labeled to have score "0". The values were summed to produce a food insecurity index. The index of food insecurity is defined as the number of items with a positive answer. The index was dichotomized as "food insecure" for adolescents having a value of 1 and above and "food secure" for those who had a value of 0. The index has high internal consistency (Cronbach's Alpha=0.81), which is above the cut off for reliability [25].

All data on background characteristics, height, and food insecurity were collected at the baseline survey. Height was repeated in the subsequent two rounds of the survey, which were conducted one year apart. Heights of adolescents were measured to the nearest 0.1 cm by trained 12 grade complete data collectors using a stadiometer (SECA, Hannover Germany). The height of each adolescent was measured without shoes. Height for age z-scores were calculated using WHO Anthro-Plus software [26].

We used repeated measures of adolescent food insecurity and height over the 2 follow up surveys and background characteristics from the baseline survey including: place of residence, household income and baseline height for age z-scores as predictor variables. Household income was divided into tertiles coded as "high", "middle" and "low".

At each round of the survey the data collection was conducted from August to February. Data collectors were interviewed at similar season of the previous survey as the data collection process was organized in a cyclic and regular manner defining the movement from one study site to the other.

5.2.3   Statistical Analyses

Data were analyzed using SAS version 9.2. The anthropometric data were checked for normality and outliers. First, exploratory analyses were carried out to identify average and subject specific evolution of height over time. The subject specific profile plots suggested that the height of adolescents varied at baseline as well as over time for each subject implying presence of considerable between and within variation. As the repeated measurements of heights taken from each subject over time are correlated, the commonly used methods like linear regression are not appropriate. There is a need for models which can take the correlation into account, combining both the fixed and random effects. To examine differences in heights within individual subjects over the follow up period, a mixed effects(fixed effects and random effects) model with a random intercept and a random slope was fitted with restricted maximum likelihood estimation method using the procedure 'proc mixed'. The fixed effects describe a population intercept and population slopes for a set of covariates, which include exposures and potential confounders. Random effects describe individual variability in height and changes over time. By considering individual random slopes and intercepts, this model allows to examine the influence of covariates on the change in height over time.

Based on stepwise likelihood ratio test, food insecurity and baseline height for age z-score, time (round of follow-up), age at baseline, household income and place of residence were used as covariates in the mean structure. To determine within subjects effect (growth over time), we included an interaction term of time of follow up with food insecurity, household income and place of residence in the models, while the main effects were used to show the effects at baseline.

Because of the correlated nature of the data, a correlation structure was specified for the measures within individuals. Some commonly used structures, namely, compound symmetric and unstructured, were used to model the covariance structure of repeated measures within subjects. We used unstructured variance matrix for girls, and compound symmetry variance (CS) matrix structure for boys as parameters of the random intercept could not be estimable due to over parameterization in the case of boys.

We stratified the analysis by sex as we expected differences in linear growth between boys and girls. As the growth of boys was not linear, we considered the quadratic effect of the time of follow up in the models. The introduction of the main quadratic time effect into the model improved the model fit based on the maximum likelihood ratio test. However, the interaction of the quadratic time effects with other covariates such as food insecurity, place of residence and income did not have any significant effect on the model fit and hence dropped from the model. All tests were two-sided and $P<0.05$ was considered statistically significant. We report the parameter estimates and standard errors (SE).

The study was approved by the Ethical Review Boards of both Brown University (USA) and Jimma University (Ethiopia). Informed verbal consent was obtained both from the parents and each respondent before the interview or measurement as approved by the ethical review committees which followed and documented the study process through supervisory visits.

5.3 RESULTS

Overall, a total of 1431 adolescents were followed for three rounds that are one year apart spanning a total follow up period of two years starting 2005. Nearly half (49.2%) were females and the rest (50.8%) were males at baseline. Analysis of socio-demographic characteristics by food security status at baseline is presented in Table 1. It was observed the proportion of food insecure adolescents was significantly high among urban adolescents (23.5%) compared to (20.2%) in the semi-urban areas and 17.9% in the rural areas (P=0.028). Similarly, the proportion of food insecure adolescents was 23% and 21.8%, respectively for low and middle income tertiles compared to 16.8% for high income tertile (P<0.001).

TABLE 5.1 Association between food security and socio-demographic variables at baseline

Variables	n	Food security status		P
		Food secure (n=1656)	Food insecure (n=428)	
Age(years)				
13	458	76.2	23.8	0.184
14	479	81.8	18.2	
15	479	81.0	19.0	
16	386	77.7	22.3	
17	282	80.4	19.6	
Place of residence				
Urban	746	76.5	23.5	0.028
Semi-Urban	589	79.8	20.2	
Rural	749	82.1	17.9	
Household income tertiles				
low	687	77.0	23.0	0.011
Middle	702	78.2	21.8	
High	695	83.2	16.8	

With regard to exposure of adolescents to food insecurity over time, 15.9% of the girls and 12.2% of the boys (P=0.018) were food insecure both at baseline and year 1 survey, while 5.5% of the girls and 4.4% of the boys (P=0.331) were food insecure in all the three rounds of the survey. In general, a significantly (P=0.045) higher proportion (40%) of girls experienced food insecurity at least in one of the survey rounds compared with boys (36.6%), Table 2.

TABLE 5.2 Baseline characteristics and repeated measures adolescents who were followed for all the three rounds of survey by sex

Characteristics	Girls	Boys	N
Adolescents Interviewed (%)			
Baseline	49.2	50.8	2084
Year 1	48.0	52.0	1911
Year 2	44.4	55.6	1431
Age of Adolescents in Years at Baseline (%)			
13	47.2	52.8	458
14	48.2	51.8	479
15	52.8	47.2	479
16	49.7	50.3	386
17	47.0	53.0	281
Place Of Residence (%)			
Urban	52.8	47.2	746
Semi-Urban	48.9	51.1	589
Rural	45.8	54.2	749
Baseline Household Income Tertile (%)			
Low	46.9	53.1	687
Middle	47.6	52.4	702
High	53.1	46.9	695
Food insecure (%)[+]			
Baseline*	$25.5(n_{1025})$*	$15.8(n_{1059})$	2084
Both baseline and year 1	$15.9(n_{917})$*	$12.2(n_{994})$	1911
All the 3 rounds	5.5(n635)	$4.4(n_{796})$	1431
At least in one of the 3 rounds	$40(n_{635})$*	36.6(n796)	1431
Mean (±SD) height (cm)			
Baseline	154.0(7.7)	157.3(11.7)	2084
Year 1	156.9(6.8)	161.5(10.8)	1911
Year 2	158.9(5.7)	169.8(7.0)	1431
Mean (±SD) HAZ[©] for age z-score at baseline	−0.91(.99)	−1.05(1.2)	2084

[+]The percentages refer to only those who are food insecure and are calculated from sex specific column totals for each follow up year.

[f]Adolescents who were food insecure at least in one of the rounds of the three surveys.

*$P<0.05$, SD = Standard Deviation.

[©]Height for age Z- Score.

As presented in Table 3, analysis of the trend of food insecurity over the follow period showed doubling of the proportion of adolescents with food insecurity from the baseline (20.5% to 48.4%) on the year 1 survey, which decreased to 27.1% during the year 2 survey.

TABLE 5.3   Trend of food insecurity and proportion of adolescents with height for age z-scores below −1 by food security and round of follow up

Variables	Food insecurity status		P	Total
	Food secure n (%)	Food insecure n (%)		
Round of survey				
Baseline	1656(79.5)	428(20.5)	<0.001	2084
Year 1	987(51.6)	924(48.4)		1911
Year 2	1043(72.9)	388(27.1)		1431
Height for age below -1Z score of the WHO reference				
Baseline				
Yes	747(46.1)	198(49.3)	0.260	915
No	838(53.9)	204(50.7)		1042
Year 1				
Yes	419(44.7)	435(50.8)	0.010	854
No	519(53.3)	422(49.2)		941
Year 2				
Yes	496(47.4)	176(45.0)	0.430	672
No	551(52.6)	215(55.0)		766

Figure 1 shows the average baseline heights of adolescent boys by age and baseline food security status compared to the WHO references for their age. Food insecure boys had their mean height on average 2.22 cm below the heights corresponding to −1SD of the WHO reference for their age, while food secure boys had mean height on average 0.32 cm below the heights corresponding to −1SD of the WHO reference. Similarly, as shown in Figure 2, the mean baseline heights of food insecure girls was on average 1.16 cm below the heights corresponding to −1SD of the WHO reference, while that of food secure girls was 1.26 cm above the heights corresponding to −1SD of the WHO reference.

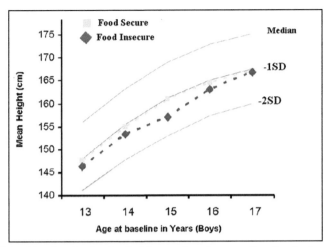

FIGURE 5.1   Mean baseline height of adolescents boys by age and baseline food security status compared to the WHO reference.

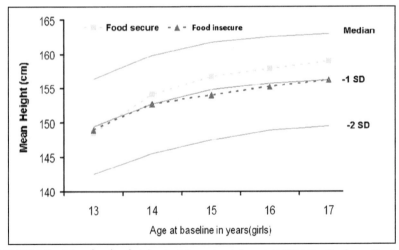

FIGURE 5.2   Mean baseline height of adolescent girls by age and baseline food security status compared to the WHO reference.

The average growth of adolescents over the three follow-up surveys is shown in Figure 3. Both food insecure boys and girls had shorter height than their food secure counterparts at all three measurements. In both boys and girls, the difference between food secure and food insecure decreased over the years although it did not disappear fully.

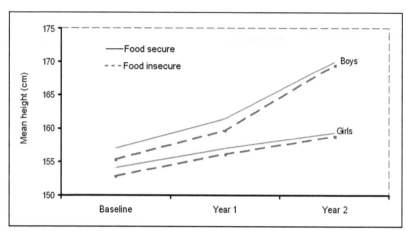

FIGURE 5.3   Growths of adolescents over the two years follow up period by food security status and sex.

As presented in Table 4, linear mixed effects model showed that food insecurity was negatively associated with height of girls baseline (ß= −0.87, P<0.0001). At baseline, food insecure girls were on average shorter by 0.87 centimeters (cms) compared with food secure girls after controlling for demographic and economic covariates. However, over the follow up period, food insecure girls grew on average by 0.38 cms more per year than food secure girls (ß =0.38, P=0.0663). Other factors positively associated with growth among girls were time (follow up year) and age at baseline. On average, when girls differed with an age of 1 year at baseline, their mean heights differed by 3.57 cms at baseline (ß =3.57, P<0.001). The height of girls increased by 3.44 cms for a unit increase in the follow up year (ß =3.44, P<0.001).

While place of residence did not have any effect on the baseline heights of girls, there was a significant difference in their growth by place of residence over the follow up period.

Compared to urban girls, the growth rate of rural girls was greater by 1.18 cms for a unit increase in the follow up year (P<0.0001), while, those in the semi-urban areas grew by 0.92 cms more for a unit increase in the follow up year compared to urban girls (P=0.0015), after adjusting for all covariates. Baseline height for age z-score was also positively associated with growth in girls (P<0.0001). For a unit increase in baseline height for age z-score, the height of girls increased by 7.39 cms on average.

TABLE 5.4 Parameter estimates and standard errors from linear mixed effects model predicting linear growth (height increase) of girls over the follow up period

Effect (n=1431)	Estimate	SE	P
Fixed Effects			
Intercept	110.260	0.9641	<.0001
Food Insecurity	−0.8689	0.1907	<.0001
Food Insecurity x Time	0.3750	0.2040	0.0663
Height for age z-scores at baseline	7.3941	0.0758	<.0001
Time	3.4408	0.2325	<.0001
Age of girls at baseline	3.5715	0.0627	<.0001
Household Income Tertile			
High (Reference)			
Middle	0.2259	0.2193	0.3032
Middle x time	0.4781	0.2993	0.1105
Low	0.6734	0.2275	0.0031
low x time	0.2218	0.3090	0.4729
Place of Residence			
Urban (Reference)			
Semi-urban	0.2694	0.2109	0.2016
Semi-urban x time	0.9145	0.2877	0.0015
Rural	0.2242	0.2228	0.3146
Rural x Time	1.1813	0.3007	<.0001
Random effects			
Variance of Random Intercept	2.9134	0.5852	
Variance of Random Slope	13.9245	0.7515	
Covariance of Random Intercept and Slope 5.6652	0.5789		
Variance of measurement errors (residuals)	12.0751	0.4551	

Restricted maximum likelihood (REML) method was used in estimating the parameters.
SE = Standard error.
Time = follow up rounds.

Results of linear mixed effects model for boys (Table 5) showed that on average when boys differed with an age of 1 year at baseline, their mean heights differed by 3.95 cms (ß=3.95, P<0.001). Food insecurity did not have a significant effect on the height of boys both baseline (ß=−0.34, P=0.3210) and over the follow up period (ß =0.14, P=0.6249). At baseline, food insecure boys were on average shorter by 0.34 centimeters (cms) after controlling for all other covariates. However, over the follow up period, food insecure boys grew by 0.14 cms more per year than food secure boys.

TABLE 5.5   Parameter estimates and standard errors from linear mixed effects model predicting linear growth (height increase) of boys over the follow up period

Effect (n=1431)	Estimate	SE	P
Fixed Effects			
Food Insecurity	−0.3382	0.3405	0.3210
Height for age z-scores at baseline	6.6557	0.0911	<.0001
Food Insecurity X Time	0.1420	0.2904	0.6249
Time	1.3737	0.4000	0.0006
Age of boys at baseline	3.9514	0.0804	<.0001
Household Income Tertile			
High (Reference)			
Middle	−0.3571	0.3695	0.3343
Middle X time	0.6131	0.3522	0.0822
Low	0.1416	0.3864	0.7140
low X time	−0.1378	0.3663	0.7069
Place of Residence			
Urban (Reference)			
Semi-urban	−0.3955	0.3546	0.2651
Semi-urban X time	0.9695	0.3396	0.0040
Rural	−0.6366	0.3717	0.0873
Rural X Time	1.1587	0.3546	0.0011
Quadratic time effect (Time2)	1.9663	0.1565	<.0001
Random effects			
Variance	14.6274	1.5378	
CS	−5.1433	0.8679	
Variance of measurement errors (residuals)	11.4764	0.4959	

Restricted maximum likelihood (REML) method was used in estimating the parameters.
Compound symmetry (CS) variance matrix structure was used to avoid over parameterization of the estimates.
SE= Standard error.
Time = follow up rounds.

Other factors that were positively associated with growth among boys were time (follow up year) and baseline height for age z-score. Over the follow up years, the height of boys increased by 1.37 cms for a unit increase in the follow up year (ß =1.37, P<0.0001). Similarly, for a unit increase in the height for age z-score at baseline, height of boys increased by 6.66 cms (ß =6.66, p<0.001).

As the mean growth plot of boys over the follow up period did not follow a linear pattern, we used a quadratic time effect in the model which was positively associated with growth (ß =1.97, P<0.0001). Introduction of the quadratic time effect into the model improved the model fit significantly (P<0.001) based on the likelihood ratio test.

Similar to the pattern observed in girls, boys had also different trajectory of growth by residence. Over the follow up period, for a unit increase in the follow up year, rural boys grew by 1.16 cms per year than their peers in the urban areas (P<0.001), while semi-urban boys grew 0.97 cms taller per year than their urban peers (P=0.004).

5.4   DISCUSSION

This study longitudinally examined the effect of food insecurity on linear growth of adolescents in the southwest Ethiopia, where food insecurity is a pervasive phenomenon [9–11]. We found that food insecure girls were shorter by nearly 1 cm (0.87 cm) compared with secure girls at baseline. Reports from the same cohort also showed that girls suffered from chronic food insecurity [9, 11], morbidity [15] school absenteeism [27] and low dietary diversity more than their boy counterparts. The fact that food insecurity was associated with a significant negative effect on the baseline height of girls might be related to male biased intra-household buffering of adolescents from food insecurity. A similar male gender bias in the intra-household distribution of food and other resources have been reported from Ethiopia [9] and other developing countries [28–31] indicating that girls are less favored in the resource constrained environments.

Food insecurity through its effect on adequate nutrient intake could hinder occurrence of catch up growth to rectify the height deficits accrued from childhood. In a food insecure situation, adolescents use food based coping strategies to survive with food shocks. These coping strategies could range from the reversible insurance strategies such as consuming low quality cheap foods, reducing the size or frequency of consumption, searching for food in socially unacceptable ways and food anxiety [23, 32]. Use of any of the coping strategies could play against the nutrient intakes of adolescents potentially leading to growth retardation. Poor dietary practices in food constrained situations are related to dietary behaviors adapted in response to food shortages [32, 33]. Stunted growth had been reported to be associated with poor dietary practices [2, 4, 5].

Recent research findings, in Guatemala indicated that stunting in early childhood can have long-term effects on cognitive development, school achievement, and economic productivity in adulthood and maternal reproductive outcomes [34]. Adolescence is the last chance for catch up of linear growth to achieve genetic potential in height [35, 36]. As a result of this rapid growth, adolescents need better nutritional care. Adverse circumstance such as food insecurity during this period would interfere the occurrence of catch up growth leading to a short adult stature. This shortness is associated with poor physical and intellectual productivity in both boys and girls. It was documented that 1% decrease in height leads to 1.4% decrease in productivity [37–39]. Empirical evidences from Ethiopia also showed that nutritional status affects agricultural productivity in adults [40]. In this study, food insecurity had significant negative effect on the growth especially in girls. Short girls are likely to have difficulties with labor and child birth [41]. In the long run, they are also likely to have low birth weight babies which will growth below the standard closing the loop of intergenerational of cycle of malnutrition [42].

Stunting during childhood can be reversed with appropriate interventions [43]. There is a potential that children who suffered childhood stunting could show catch up growth [35, 44] although it is not a complete catch up as a complete catch growth may require trans-generational catch-up [44]. A study from Senegal reported that children stunted during childhood caught up with their genetic potential, although the height difference between stunted and nonstunted children continued to persist [35]. It has been shown that the four phases of human growth (fetal, infancy childhood and pubertal) are interlinked. Inadequate height gain during the childhood phase may trigger more height gain during the puberty phase and catch-up growth during puberty is likely to occur if the child has experienced malnutrition in childhood [44, 45]. Our results showed that regardless of the faster growth of food insecure girls and boys during the two years follow up period, they did not catch up their food secure peers indicating that the catch up growth is not adequate. Unlike the catch up growth in younger children (Type A), where the growth increases up to 4 times the mean growth velocity for chronological age, the type of catch up growth that occurs during adolescence is type B, where a delay in growth and somatic development persists when growth restriction ceases and growth continues for longer than usual to compensate for the growth deficit [46]. However, in this study, we used adolescents who were 13–17 years who had already elapsed their growth spurt ages, especially in the case of girls [1, 2], which is one of our limitations. Despite the fact that growth might continue for longer period to compensate for growth deficits of food insecure adolescents, the fact that they are already beyond the age of growth spurt, the slow increase in height in Type B catch up growth and the pervasive nature of food insecurity in the study community may jeopardize the possibility of full catch up in both boys and girls.

Adult short stature results from nutritional deficit at the different phases of growth rather than just in a single phase [45]. Evidence shows that children with faster linear growth in infancy and childhood had less height gain between ages during adolescence [45, 47]. Childhood stunting is highly prevalent in Ethiopia [19, 48] and the last chance for curbing the consequences of malnutrition on linear growth is adolescence period. Our results imply that in food insecure situations, adolescents need to be targeted in nutrition programs in addition to intervention that are in place during early childhood to promote catch up growth and prevent them form growing into an adult with a short stature. Chronic malnutrition during early childhood is responsible for widespread stunting and adverse health and social consequences throughout the life span. Although this is best prevented during childhood [44] to improve access to food could benefit adolescents as well. Key interventions to promote adolescent growth such as prevention of anemia through iron supplementation and or deworming, school feeding programs and prevention of teenage pregnancy and improving the nutritional status of girls before they enter pregnancy could help to break the intergenerational cycle of malnutrition [49]. In addition to the above, food security intervention targeting adolescents' should be considered.

For both boys and girls, adolescents in the rural and in the semi-urban areas grew more per years than those in the urban areas. This might be related to the lower frequency of food insecurity prevailing in these areas compared to the urban areas as presented in Table 1.

This study used longitudinal data to demonstrate the effect of food insecurity on growth of adolescents. We acknowledge limitations in interpreting the results of this study. During the follow up period, large number of adolescents was lost to follow up (31.3% of the baseline sample), although this has been taken into consideration during the sample size calculation. We considered in our analyses if this attrition has affected the results in an important way. Most of the adolescents lost were females and older age groups and there was no difference in baseline food insecurity between adolescents that are still in the study and those who were lost to follow up (19.5% VS 22.5%, P=0.081). Entering the effect of adolescents lost to follow up into the multivariable model showed that there was no significant effect in the results. Use of self reported food insecurity questions could also lead to social desirability biases. However as the food security scales are validated in developing countries, it is expected that this problem is minimal. Errors during anthropometric measurements are also possible and could lead to measurement bias. However, in this study, the data collectors were intensively trained on anthropometric measurement procedures and they were also supervised during data collection.

5.5 CONCLUSIONS

Food insecurity is negatively associated with the linear growth of adolescents, especially on girls. Although on average food insecure boys and girls grew faster over the follow up period, they did not catch with their food secure peers at the end of the two years follow up indicating that the catch up is not adequate. The results indicate that as catch up growth takes longer time, food insecure adolescents towards the end of their growth years may not be able to catch up. High prevalence of childhood stunting in Ethiopia compounded with the negative effect of food insecurity on adolescents growth calls for the development of direct nutrition interventions targeting adolescents to promote faster catch-up growth and break the intergenerational cycle of malnutrition. Inadequate growth (stunting) is the reflection of socioeconomic development demanding combination of different types of policies and programmes for its solution. Strategies for reducing and preventing stunting need to involve a combination of macro-economic policies and more targeted interventions. Promoting gender equality and the status of women and girls through effective behavior change communications at grassroots level needs to be considered. Further research will help to understand these linkages as a way to identify the most effective strategies for reducing adolescent malnutrition in the socio-cultural environment of the study community.

REFERENCES

1. Tanner JM, Whitehouse RH, Marshall WA, Carter BS: Prediction of adult height, bone age, and occurrence of menarche, at age 4 to 16 with allowance for mid parental height. Arch Dis Child 1975, 50:14–26.
2. Rogol AD, Roemmich JN, Clark PA: Growth at Puberty. J Adolesc Health 2002, 31:192–200.
3. Mustanski BS, Viken RJ, Kaprio J, Pulkkinen L, Rose RJ: Genetic and environmental influences on pubertal development: longitudinal data from Finnish twins at ages 11 and 14. Dev Psychol 2004,40(6):1188–1198.
4. Berkey CS, Gardner JD, Frazier AL, Colditz GA: Relation of childhood diet and body size to menarche and adolescent growth in girls. Am J Epidemiol 2000 Sep 1,152(5):446–452.
5. Berkey CS, Colditz GA, Rockett HR, Frazier AL, Willett WC: Dairy consumption and female height growth: prospective cohort study. Cancer Epidemiol Biomarkers Prev 2009 Jun,18(6):1881–1887.

6. Biro FM, Lucky AW, Simbartl LA: Pubertal maturation in girls and the relationship to anthropometric changes: pathways through puberty. J Pediatr 2003 Jun,142(6):643–646.

7. Cheng G, Gerlach S, Libuda L, Kranz S: Diet quality in childhood is prospectively associated with the timing of puberty but not with body composition at puberty onset. J Nutr 2010,140(1):95–102.

8. Rogol AD, Clark PA, Roemmich JN: Growth and pubertal development in children and adolescents: effects of diet and physical activity. Am J Clin Nutr 2000 Aug,72(2 Suppl):521S-528S.

9. Hadley C, Lindstrom D, Tessema F, Belachew T: Gender bias in food insecurity experiences of adolescents in Jimma zone. Soc SciMed. 2008,66(2):427–438.

10. Hadley C, Belachew T, Lindstrom D, Tessema F: The forgotten population? Youth, food insecurity, and rising prices: implications for the global food crisis. NAPA Bull. 2009, 32:77–91.

11. Belachew T, Lindstrom D, Gebremariam A: Predictors of chronic food insecurity among adolescents in Southwest Ethiopia: a longitudinal study. BMC Publ Health 2012 Aug 3, 12:604.

12. Chilton M, Chyatte M, Breaux J: The negative effects of poverty & food insecurity on child development. Indian J Med Res 2007 Oct,126(4):262–272.

13. Cook JT, Frank DA, Levenson SM: Child food insecurity increases risks posed by household food insecurity to young children's health. J Nutr 2006 Apr,136(4):1073–1076.

14. Kirkpatrick SI, McIntyre L, Potestio ML: Child hunger and long-term adverse consequences for health. Arch Pediatr Adolesc Med 2010 Aug,164(8):754–762.

15. Belachew T, Haley C, Lindtsrom D: Gender differences in food insecurity and morbidity among adolescents in southwest Ethiopia. Pediatrics 2011,127(2):e397-e404.

16. Widome R, Neumark-Sztainer D, Hannan PJ, Haines J, Story M: Eating when there is not enough to eat: eating behaviors and perceptions of food among food-insecure youths. Am J Public Health 2009 May,99(5):822–828.

17. Loth K, van den Berg P, Eisenberg ME, Neumark-Sztainer D: Stressful life events and disordered eating behaviors: findings from Project EAT. J Adolesc Health 2008 Nov,43(5):514–516.

18. Kolsteren PW, Kusin JA, Sri K: Pattern of linear growth velocities of children from birth to 12 months in Madura, Indonesia. J Trop Med Int Health 1997,2(3):291–301.

19. Central Statistical Agency Addis Ababa. Ethiopia & ORC Macro: Ethiopia demographic and health survey; 2011.

20. Mulugeta A, Hagos F, Stoecker B: Nutritional status of adolescent girls from rural communities of Tigray, Northern Ethiopia. Ethiop J Health Dev 2009,23(1):5–11.

21. Kish L: A procedure for objective respondent selection within the household. Jam Stat Assoc 1949, 44:380–387.

22. Coates J, Frongillo EA, Rogers BL, Swindale A, Bilinsky P: Measuring household food insecurity: why it's so important and yet so difficult to do? J Nutr 2006, 136:1404S-1408Sa.

23. Coates J, Frongillo EA, Rogers BL, Webb P, Wilde PE, House R: Commonalities in the experience of household food insecurity across cultures: what are measures missing? J Nutr 2006, 136:1438S-1448Sb.

24. Frongillo EA, Nanama S: Development and validation of an experience-based measure of household food security within and across seasons in northern Burkina Faso. J Nutr 2006,136(5):1409S-1419S.

25. Nunnally JC: Psychometric theory. 2nd edition. New York: McGraw-Hill; 1978.

26. WHO: AnthroPlus for personal computers Manual: Software for assessing growth of the world's children and adolescents. Geneva: WHO; 2009. (Available from: http://www.who. int/growthref/en/) [Accessed on November 1, 2011]

27. Belachew T, Hadley C, Lindstrom D, Gebremariam A, Lachat C, Kolsteren P: Food insecurity, school absenteeism and educational attainment: a longitudinal study. Nutr J 2011, 10:29.

28. Senauer B, Garcia M, Jacinto E: Determinants of the intra-household allocation of food in the rural Philippines. Am J Agric Econ 1988,70(1):170–180.

29. Behrman J: Intra-household allocation of nutrients in Rural India: are boys favored? Do parents exhibit inequality aversion? Oxf Econ Pap 1988,40(1):32–54.

30. Gittelsohn J, Thapa M, Landman LT: Cultural factors, caloric intake and micronutrient sufficiency in rural Nepali households. Soc Sci Med 1997,44(11):1739–1749.

31. Frongillo EA Jr, Begin F: Gender bias in food intake favors male preschool Guatemalan children. J Nutr 1993,123(2):189–196.

32. Norhasmah S, Zalilah MS, Mohd Nasir MT, Kandiah M, Asnarulkhadi AS: A qualitative study on coping strategies among women from food insecurity households in Selangor and Negeri Sembilan. Mal J Nutr 2010,16(1):39–54.

33. Hamelin A-M, Habicht J-P, Beaudry M: Food Insecurity: consequences for the household and broader social implications. J Nutr 1999, 129:525S-528S.

34. Dewey KG, Begum K: Long-term consequences of stunting in early life. Matern Child Nutr 2011,7(Suppl. 3):5–18.

35. Coly AN, Milet J, Diallo A: Preschool stunting, adolescent migration, catch-up growth, and adult height in young Senegalese men and women of rural origin. J Nutr 2006 Sep,136(9):2412–2420.

36. Eisenstein E: Chronic under Nutrition During adolescence. Ann N Y Acad Sci 2006,817(1):138–161.

37. Haddad L, Bouis H: The Impact of Nutritional Status on Agricultural Productivity: Wage Evidence from the Philippines. Oxford Bulletin of Economic Studies 1990,53(1):45–68.

38. WHO: Adolescent Nutrition at a glance. 2003. http://siteresources.worldbank.org/ INTPHAAG/Resources/AAGAdolNutrEng.pdf [Accessed on November 1, 2011]

39. Thomas D, Strauss J: Health and wages: Evidence on men and women in urban Brazil. J Econ 1997, 77:159–185.

40. Croppenstedt A, Muller C: The impact of farmers' health and nutritional status on their productivity and efficiency: Evidence from Ethiopia. Econ Dev Cult Chang April 2000,48(3):475–502.

41. Konje JC, Ladipo OA: Nutrition and obstructed labor. Am J Clin Nutr 2000 Jul,72(1 Suppl):291S-297S.

42. Ramakrishnan U, Martorell R, Schroeder DG, Flores R: Role of intergenerational effects on linear growth. J Nutr 1999 Feb,129(2S Suppl):544S-549S.

43. IJzendoorn MH, Juffer F: The Emanuel Miller Memorial Lecture 2006: Adoption as intervention. Meta-analytic evidence for massive catch-up and plasticity in physical, socio-emotional, and cognitive development. J Child Psychol Psychiatry 2006,47(12):1228–1245.

44. Golden MHN: Is complete catch-up possible for stunted malnourished children? Eur J Clin Nutr 1994,48(Supplement):S58-S71.

45. Luo ZC, Karlberg J: Critical Growth Phases for Adult Shortness. Am J Epidemiol 2000, 152:125–131.

46. Boersma B, Wit JN: Catch-up Growth. Endocr Rev 1997,18(5):646–661.

47. Luo ZC, Cheung YB, He Q, Albertsson-Wikland K, Karlberg J: Growth in early life and its relation to pubertal growth. Epidemiology 2003 Jan,14(1):65–73.

48. Central Statistical Agency Addis Ababa. Ethiopia & ORC Macro: Ethiopia demographic and health survey 2005; 2006.

49. Nestel P: Strategies, Policies and Programs to Improve the Nutrition of Women and Girls. FANTA; 2000. http://www.fantaproject.org/downloads/pdfs/StrategiesPoliciesPrograms_ Nestel.pdf

Factors Associated with Stunting Among Children According to the Level of Food Insecurity in the Household: A Cross-Sectional Study in a Rural Community of Southeastern Kenya

Chisa Shinsugi, Masaki Matsumura,
Mohamed Karama, Junichi Tanaka,
Mwatasa Changoma, and Satoshi Kaneko

6.1 BACKGROUND

Child malnutrition is still one of the most serious health problems in countries in sub-Saharan Africa and South Asia. It is estimated that nearly 3.1 million children die annually either directly or indirectly as a result of malnutrition [1], and approximately 165 million children are affected by chronic restriction of potential growth [2]. Damage to growth in the early years of life is largely irreversible in terms of human capital development [3-5].

Stunting (low height-for-age) is the chronic restriction of a child's potential growth. Specifically, it refers to children from the ages of 0 to 59 months who are below 2 standard deviations from the median height-for-age determined by the World Health Organization (WHO) Child Growth Standards [6,7]. Along with wasting (low weight-for-height) and underweight (low weight-for-age), stunting is an indicator of undernutrition. As shown in the conceptual model from UNICEF [8,9], causal factors for stunting in children under 5 years old vary with age and are ecologically linked with each other. Among them, environmental factors in households, i.e., household food security and healthy household environment, play important roles in preventing stunting in the longer term [10-13]. The household environment related to child nutrition consists of the perception by caregivers of food insecurity [14], child health and food selection [15-17], and household socioeconomic status [18]. These intra-household environmental factors contribute to the neglect of children's needs, especially their nutritional status from birth to preschool. Furthermore, the intra-household environment is affected by environmental, cultural, and historical factors in the communities where the mothers live.

Although the proportion of children with stunted growth has declined from 35% in 2000 to 30% in 2008 to 2009 [19], Kenya is one of 34 countries with the highest burden of child malnutrition in the world [1]. This study was designed to examine the influence of household environmental factors on the nutritional status of children under 5 years old in a community with a high level of food insecurity in rural Kenya, with the aim of seeking solutions at the community level to ameliorate the problem of childhood stunting.

6.2 METHODS

A cross-sectional study was conducted in Kwale District in the Coast Province of Kenya in 2012, using a cohort nested to the Health and Demographic Surveillance System (HDSS) program, which follows about 50,000 residents periodically, in collaboration with Nagasaki University and the Kenya Medical Research Institute [20]. In this cohort, we recruited children under 5 years old and their caregivers, including non-biological mothers, from households located within a radius of 2.2 km from the Kizibe Health Center, one of the health centers in the HDSS program area. The radius was set in consideration of accessibility for children and their caregivers to the surveys in the nested-cohort study. We took into consideration the estimated sampling size (438 children) for a 2 sample comparison of proportions calculated in the study design stage assuming that 10% of children would become stunted during the observation period and there would be twice as many children with stunting in the comparison group, which has a factor (exposure) with a power of 80% and a significance level of 5% (2-tailed). This cohort program measured several indices, including anthropometric measurements such as height and weight, and asked questions of mothers related to health status and dietary intake. The measurements were to take place 3 times per year between 2011 and 2014. In this cross-sectional study, a structured questionnaire was additionally administered as part of the follow-up surveys of the cohort to investigate the relationship between intra-household environment and child nutritional status. During the survey period in 2012, 653 households were registered within a 2.2-km radius from the health center of the HDSS program; and among them, 516 children less than 5 years old were identified in 360 households.

After carrying out a pre-test to revise the questionnaire for suitability, we conducted interviews of the caregivers by trained local investigators in the Kiswahili language at the health center. The interview required approximately 20 minutes to complete. The structured questionnaire consisted of the following variables: demographic characteristics; socioeconomic status; household food security; child health status, such as breastfeeding behavior and illness in the past 2 weeks including jigger flea (Tunga penetrans) infection; caregiver's perception of child's growth; and caregiver's household chores as a proximal factor of availability for child rearing.

The household food security level was measured using the Household Food Insecurity Access Scale (HFIAS) with scores ranging from 0 to 27 by household level [21]. The HFIAS scores obtained from households were categorized into 4 levels of food insecurity, namely, "food secure," "mildly food insecure," "moderately food insecure," and "severely food insecure," based on the HFIAS guideline [22]. The household socioeconomic status (SES) was parameterized by the principle component analysis (PCA) method using house properties confirmed by the questionnaire: property owned; source of drinking water; type of toilet facility; and type of flooring, wall material, and roof material. The items of household property were selected according to the Demographic Health Survey (DHS) [19]. The score in the first PCA component was used as an asset index of SES status for each household [23]. According to the PCA-based asset index, households were divided into 4 groups; the first quartile SES group was poorest and the fourth quartile SES group was richest in the study area.

For data validation, Cronbach's alpha coefficient, which is a measure of the internal consistency of a scale, was used to confirm the reliability of the HFIAS and household SES measure. An alpha value of more than 0.7 indicates that the measure is acceptable. Child age was confirmed using his/her maternal and child health (MCH) handbook or by the response from the caregiver if the MCH handbook was not available.

Anthropometric measurement data were obtained from the child cohort dataset. In the child cohort study, height was measured by a length scale (Seca GmbH & Co.Kg, Germany). Weight was measured using trouser for baby weighing scale (G.S.T. Corporation, India) and portable electronic scale (Guangzhou Weiheng Electronics Co., Ltd, China) for babies; and KRUPS Baby Cum Child Weighing Scale (Doctor Beci Ram & Sons [MFG.], India) for children who could stand. For measuring the weight of caregivers a Tanita THD-650 scale (Tanita, Japan) was used.

Chronic malnutrition (stunting) of children was defined as z-score below 2 standard deviations(SD) from the mean for length or height for age according to the Child Growth Standards published by the WHO in 2006 [6]. For this study, those who had a z-score above −2 SD were defined as children who did not have stunting.

We excluded the following children from the analysis: those whose caregivers were unable to answer the questions due to hearing disability; those who were severely sick; and those whose birth date were not appropriate or unclear. Because 72.3% of children in this study were born at home according to our survey data, some birth dates were not clearly recorded.

The association between potential predictors (child and caregiver characteristics, intra-household environment, food intake, and health history) and stunting status was determined by univariate logistic regression analyses. Because some children belong to the same household and may be correlated, cluster options by household were incorporated in the logistic regression. Multiple logistic regression analysis was also conducted to control confounding factors by backward stepwise selection with 0.2 of significant level of removal from the model as well as cluster option by household. Additionally, to identify associated factors of childhood stunting separately in severe and non-severe food insecurity groups, the analyses were independently conducted for the 2 groups in the same statistical manner. Stata statistical software (version 12.0: Stata Corporation, TX, USA) was used for data cleansing and data analyses.

This study was approved by the Ethics Committee of Nagasaki University and authorized as a sub-study of the cohort study by the Ethical Review Committee of the Kenya Medical Research Institute (KEMRI SSC No.1964). Study permission was also obtained from the National Council for Science and Technology

(NCST) in Kenya (Research Permit No. NCST/RCD/12A/012/59). We explained the study objectives and obtained written informed consent from all participants before collecting data. Participants were informed that participation in this study was voluntary and that they could stop participating at any time without experiencing negative consequences.

6.3   RESULTS

Four hundred twenty-five selected children were initially enrolled in this study. Twenty-one children were excluded (severely sick, 2; no or inadequate date of birth, 17; and hearing disability of caregiver, 2). Finally, 404 children less than 5 years old from 263 households participated in the survey conducted at the health center. The response rate was 78.3% (404/516). Among the remaining children, 94 (23.3%) were stunted and 310 (76.7%) were not stunted according to WHO child growth standards [6]. The distributions of height-for-age of the children are presented in Figure 1 along with the WHO standards.

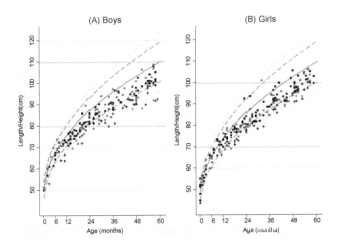

FIGURE 6.1   Distributions of length/height-for-age from birth to 59 months: (A): Boys, (B): Girls. The 5 lines represent median (solid green line) and standard deviations (SD) from the median length/height-for-age provided by the World Health Organization Child Growth Standards: +/−3 SD (dotted gray line), +/−2 SD (dashed orange line) between median and +/−3 SD lines. Black circles: children without stunting in the severe food insecure group; black +: children with stunting in the severe food insecure group; red triangle: children without stunting in the non-severe food insecure group; red x: children with stunting in the non-severe food insecure group.

In Table 1, characteristics of the children and their families are displayed according to stunting status of children and crude odds ratios (ORs). Children aged 12 months and older were significantly more likely to be stunted compared with children less than 6 months old. Forty (21.5%) boys and 54 (24.8%) girls were determined to have stunted growth; but there was no significant difference between boys and girls regarding stunting status. There were 263 caregivers for 404 children and the mean age of caregivers was 29.2 years old (standard deviation [SD]: 7.9; range: 14–72). Children who had adolescent caregivers or caregivers more than 40 years old were more likely to be stunted, but this was not statistically significant. The mean body mass index (BMI) of caregivers was 20.7 kg/m^2 (range: 13.9-37.5). Ninety-eight (24.5%) caregivers were underweight (BMI < 18.5 kg/m^2), but there was no significant association of childhood stunting according to category of caregiver BMI. Almost half of the caregivers had received a primary-school education, but half had not completed primary school. There was no significant difference in child stunting distribution or association according to caregiver education level. The mean number of siblings of preschool age was 1.9 per household. Children with two or more siblings of preschool age were significantly more likely to suffer from chronic malnutrition (OR: 1.69; 95% CI: 1.01-2.83).

TABLE 6.1   Distribution of stunting status by characteristics of children (N = 404)

Variables	Children with stunting		Children without stunting		Total
Child age (mo)					
0-5	3	(7.5%)	37	(92.5%)	40
6-11	6	(15.8%)	32	(84.2%)	38
12-23	21	(23.1%)	70	(76.9%)	91
24-35	21	(29.2%)	51	(70.8%)	72
36-47	24	(32.0%)	51	(68.0%)	75
48-59	19	(21.6%)	69	(78.4%)	88
Child gender					
Boy	40	(21.5%)	146	(78.5%)	186
Girl	54	(24.8%)	164	(75.2%)	218
Caregiver's age (y)					
18 and younger	5	(38.5%)	8	(61.5%)	13
19-30	51	(22.1%)	180	(77.9%)	231
31-40	29	(21.5%)	106	(78.5%)	135
Above 40	8	(34.8%)	15	(65.2%)	23
Missing	1	(50.0%)	1	(50.0%)	2

TABLE 6.1   *(Continued)*

Variables	Children with stunting		Children without stunting		Total
Caregiver's BMI					
Underweight	28	(28.6%)	70	(71.4%)	98
Normal	56	(21.0%)	211	(79.0%)	267
Overweight	7	(30.4%)	16	(69.6%)	23
Obese	3	(25.0%)	9	(75.0%)	12
Missing	0	(0.0%)	4	(100.0%)	4
Caregiver's education status					
Not educated	49	(26.2%)	138	(73.8%)	187
Preschool	0	(0.0%)	9	(100.0%)	9
Primary	44	(22.8%)	149	(77.2%)	193
Secondary	1	(6.7%)	14	(93.3%)	15
0 or 1	28	(17.8%)	129	(82.2%)	157
2 or more	66	(26.8%)	180	(73.2%)	246
Missing	0	(0.0%)	1	(100.0%)	1
HFIAS* category (food insecurity)					
Secure	15	(20.0%)	60	(80.0%)	75
Mildly insecure	6	(18.8%)	26	(81.3%)	32
Moderately insecure	7	(17.9%)	32	(82.1%)	39
Severely insecure	66	(25.6%)	192	(74.4%)	258
Socio economic status (SES)					
Poorest	31	(28.4%)	78	(71.6%)	109
Second	19	(20.7%)	73	(79.3%)	92
Third	29	(28.7%)	72	(71.3%)	101
Fourth	15	(15.0%)	85	(85.0%)	100
Missing	0	(0.0%)	2	(100.0%)	2
Child health conditions					
Diarrhea					
No	61	(22.2%)	214	(77.8%)	275
Yes	32	(25.0%)	96	(75.0%)	128
Missing	1	(100.0%)	0	(0.0%)	1
Current jiggers infection					
No	59	(20.4%)	230	(79.6%)	289
Yes	34	(29.8%)	80	(70.2%)	114
Missing	1	(100.0%)	0	(0.0%)	1

TABLE 6.1   *(Continued)*

Variables	Children with stunting		Children without stunting		Total
Ring worm					
No	69	(21.9%)	246	(78.1%)	315
Yes	24	(27.3%)	64	(72.7%)	88
Missing	1	(100.0%)	0	(0.0%)	1
Dietary intake in previous 24 h					
Plain water					
No	11	(20.0%)	44	(80.0%)	55
Yes	83	(23.8%)	266	(76.2%)	349
Non-milk liquids					
No	51	(21.3%)	189	(78.8%)	240
Yes	42	(25.8%)	121	(74.2%)	163
Missing	1	(100.0%)	0	(0.0%)	1
Tea/porridge with milk in previous 24 h					
No	58	(20.4%)	227	(79.6%)	285
Yes	35	(29.7%)	83	(70.3%)	118
Missing	1	(100.0%)	0	(0.0%)	1

*HFIAS, Household Food Insecurity Access Scale.

Prior to analyzing the relationship between household food insecurity level and child stunting, internal consistency was evaluated by Cronbach's alpha obtained for the 9 questions of the HFIAS for 263 households. Cronbach's alpha was 0.96, which indicates that internal consistency was sufficient for further analysis. A score of 0 indicates that the household does not have food insecurity, whereas a score of 27 indicates that the household has severe food insecurity. The mean HFIAS score was 9.85 (SD: 8.5; median: 9.0), with a range of 0 to 27. Among 263 households, 165 (62.7%) were categorized as having severe food insecurity. The number of moderately and mildly insecure and secure households were 29 (11.0%), 22 (8.4%), and 47 (17.9%), respectively. The association with stunting was not significantly different among the food insecure categories.

Regarding SES, the majority of participants lived in compounds consisting of natural materials with several buildings designated for cooking and housing animals. The household wealth quartile index was determined by estimating asset factors through principle component analysis (PCA). The first component of the PCA, with a 16.1% proportion, was used to determine household socio-economic status (SES) as a proxy indicator. Cronbach's alpha obtained from the 27 items measuring SES was 0.71, confirming the reliability of this scale.

Compared to the poorest category, there was no significant difference in the prevalence of stunting in the second and third SES categories. However, there was 59% less stunting in the fourth SES category (wealthiest) compared to the poorest category.

The distribution and prevalence of illnesses among the children according to the children's medical records for the previous 2 weeks are listed in Table 1. Diarrhea and jiggers and ringworm infections were included in consideration of their high morbidity in the area. One hundred twenty-eight children (31.7%) had diarrhea in the previous 2 weeks and 114 (28.2%) suffered from jiggers infection, which is an indigenous disease in resource-poor communities and has not been significantly associated with chronic malnutrition among children (OR: 1.66; 95% CI: 0.99-2.77; p = 0.055). The distribution and prevalence of children with stunting by dietary intake in the previous 24 hours are also presented in Table 1. In the previous 24 hours, the majority of children (n: 349; 86.4%) drank plain water and 163 (40.3%) drank non-milk liquids. One hundred eighteen children (29.2%) had tea/porridge with milk in the previous 24 hours and those children were 1.65 times more likely to have stunting (95% CI: 1.03-2.64; p = 0.036) compared with those who did not have tea/porridge with milk.

6.3.1 Multivariate Analysis

The results from the stepwise multiple regression model of stunted children on household and caregiver variables are shown in Table 2. The following factors remained and were incorporated into the regression model: socioeconomic status (SES), child age in months, animal rearing, number of siblings of pre-school age, having something to drink with milk in the previous 24 hours, and current jiggers infection. HFIAS category was forced into the model to evaluate the effect of food insecurity on child stunting. Among the variables remaining in the model, children in households in the highest SES category had 66% less stunting compared with those in the poorest households (OR: 0.34; 95% CI: 0.16-0.72); however, the food insecurity level (HFIAS category) was not significantly different among these groups. Children between 2 and 3 years old were about 3.5 times more likely to be stunted compared with those aged 0 to 5 months (OR: 3.58; 95% CI: 1.33-20.10 for those aged 24–35 months; OR: 3.43; 95% CI: 1.40-18.98 for those aged 36–47 months). Other factors that had tendencies of associations but were not significant were living with 2 or more siblings (preschool-age) compared with those with fewer than 2 siblings: adjusted OR [aOR]: 1.59 (95% CI: 0.93-2.73); given tea or porridge: aOR: 1.69 (95% CI: 0.98-2.93); and a current jiggers infection: aOR: 1.48 (95% CI: 0.83-2.64).

TABLE 6.2   Odds ratios (ORs) for child stunting among the whole child group using univariate and multiple logistic regressions

Variables	Crude OR	95% CI	Adjusted OR	95% CI
Child age (mo)				
0-5	Ref.		Ref.	
6-11	2.31	(0.51 - 10.42)	1.85	(0.52 - 10.89)
12-23	3.70	(1.02 - 13.45)	2.48	(0.92 - 13.95)
24-35	5.08	(1.46 - 17.69)	3.58	(1.33 - 20.10)
36-47	5.80	(1.71 - 19.75)	3.43	(1.40 - 18.98)
48-59	3.40	(0.96 - 12.02)	2.13	(0.72 - 12.10)
Child gender				
Boys	Ref.		Ref.	
Girls	1.20	(0.75 - 1.92)	1.52	(0.92 - 2.52)
Caregiver's age (y)				
18 and younger	2.21	(0.62 - 7.84)		
19-30	Ref.			
31-40	0.97	(0.56 - 1.67)		
Above 40	1.88	(0.78 - 4.53)		
Missing	-			
Caregiver's BMI				
Underweight	Ref.			
Normal	0.66	(0.40 - 1.11)		
Overweight	1.09	(0.41 - 2.94)		
Obese	0.83	(0.16 - 4.26)		
Caregiver's education status				
Not educated	Ref.			
Preschool	-			
Primary	0.83	(0.51 - 1.35)		
Secondary	0.20	(0.02 - 1.64)		
Siblings of preschool age				
0 or 1	Ref.	Ref.		
2 or more	1.69	(1.01 - 2.83)	1.59	(0.93 - 2.73)
HFIAS* category (food insecurity)				
Secure	Ref.		Ref.	
Mildly insecure	0.92	(0.29 - 2.95)	1.02	(0.30 - 3.47)

TABLE 6.2   *(Continued)*

Variables	Crude OR	95% CI	Adjusted OR	95% CI
Moderately insecure	0.88	(0.32 - 2.38)	0.94	(0.32 - 2.77)
Severely insecure	1.38	(0.70 - 2.69)	1.17	(0.56 - 2.43)
Socio economic status (SES				
Poorest	Ref.		Ref.	
Second	0.65	(0.34 - 1.26)	0.59	(0.29 - 1.17)
Third	0.80	(0.42 - 1.50)	0.68	(0.33 - 1.41)
Fourth	0.41	(0.20 - 0.82)	0.34	(0.16 - 0.72)
Child health conditions				
Diarrhea				
No	Ref.			
Yes	1.17	(0.71 - 1.93)		
Current jiggers infection				
No	Ref.		Ref.	
Yes	1.66	(0.99 - 2.77)	1.48	(0.83 - 2.64)
Ring worm				
No	Ref.			
Yes	1.34	(0.80 - 2.25)		
Dietary intake in previous 24 h				
Plain water				
No	Ref.			
Yes	1.25	(0.66 - 2.37)		
Non-milk liquids				
No	Ref.			
Yes	1.29	(0.79 - 2.08)		
Tea/porridge with milk in previous 24 h				
No	Ref.		Ref.	
Yes	1.65	(1.03 - 2.64)	1.69	(0.98 - 2.93)
Animal rearing				
No	Ref.		Ref.	
Yes	1.82	(1.06 - 3.11)	1.62	(0.87 - 3.01)

Note: 393 among 404 children with non-missing variables were used for the multivariate logistic regression analysis. For multivariate logistic regression, all variables listed in Table 1 were used and selected by backward stepwise selectin with 0.2 of significant level of removal from the model. All the selected variables were used for calculating adjusted odds ratios (adjusted ORs).
*HFIAS, Household Food Insecurity Access Scale

The factors associated with childhood stunting were also analyzed separately for food insecure household groups and groups that were not food insecure using a stepwise logistic regression model, because different factors would affect child stunting status at different food security levels. The results are shown in Table 3. In food insecure households, the significant factors associated with child stunting were tea or porridge intake (aOR: 3.22; 95% CI: 1.43-7.25), child age (those aged 24–35 months), and socioeconomic status. The factor of jigger infection remained in the model but it was not statistically significant (aOR: 1.84; 95% CI: 0.88-3.84).

TABLE 6.3   Adjusted odd ratios for child stunting among separate child groups by household food insecurity level using multiple logistic regression

Variables	Adjusted OR	95% CI
1) Severe food insecure group (N = 252)		
Tea/porridge with milk in previous 24 h		
No	Ref.	
Yes	3.22	(1.43 - 7.25)
Non-milk liquids		
No	Ref.	
Yes	0.50	(0.22 - 1.16)
Jigger infection		
No	Ref.	
Yes	1.84	(0.88 - 3.84)
Child age (mo)		
0-5	Ref.	
6-11	2.38	(0.48 - 11.92)
12-23	1.89	(0.47 - 7.62)
24-35	4.04	(1.01 - 16.14)
36-47	3.16	(0.85 - 11.79)
48-59	1.59	(0.36 - 6.94)
Socioeconomic status (SES)		
Poorest	Ref.	
Second	0.71	(0.33 - 1.53)
Third	0.80	(0.35 - 1.85)
Fourth	0.33	(0.13 - 0.85)

TABLE 6.3   *(Continued)*

Variables	Adjusted OR	95% CI
2) Non-severe food insecure group (N = 108)		
Animal rearing		
No	Ref.	
Yes	3.24	(1.04 - 10.07)
Caregiver's education status		
Not educated/Preschool	Ref.	
Primary/Secondary	0.44	(0.16 - 1.26)
Socioeconomic status (SES)		
Poorest	Ref.	
Second	0.14	(0.03 - 0.73)
Third	0.22	(0.04 - 1.08)
Fourth	0.13	(0.03 - 0.55)
Siblings of preschool age		
0 or 1	Ref.	
2 or more	2.81	(0.92 - 8.58)

Note: OR, Odds Ratio; 95% CI, 95% Confidence Interval; HFIAS, Household Food Insecurity Access Scale.

For multivariate logistic regression, all variables listed in Table 1 were used and selected by backward stepwise selection with 0.2 of significant level of removal from the model. All the selected variables were used for calculating adjusted odds ratios (adjusted ORs).

For non-severe-food insecure group, 33 children aged less than 12 months were removed from the analysis because only 1 stunting condition was found in these categories.

In non-food insecure household groups, children in households with animal rearing had a significant association with stunting (aOR: 3.24; 95% CI: 1.04-10.07). Also, socioeconomic status was significantly associated. The association with stunting for participants in the second, third, and fourth SES (wealthiest) categories was significant compared with the first category (poorest). The factor of siblings of pre-school age remained in the model, but was not significant (aOR: 2.81; 95% CI: 0.92-8.58).

6.4   DISCUSSION

This study was initially designed to evaluate the influence of the intra-household environment, especially food insecurity, on chronic malnutrition or stunting among children under 5 years old in a highly food insecure area of Kenya. This idea was initiated by the conceptual framework of the determinants of child undernutrition presented by UNICEF, which describes the relations of these environmental factors in households to stunting in children [7]. The relationships between household food insecurity and childhood stunting has been reported in some Asian and African countries, as indicated in the framework described [24-26]. However, food insecurity level was not significantly related to child stunting in this study. The discrepant result might be due to the skewed distribution of the households in our study toward the food insecurity side with a narrow range, but the real reason cannot be determined with this study design. Nonetheless, it is important to know associated factors for childhood stunting for both food insecure and food secure household groups from the public health perspective.

In households with severe food insecurity, children who had been given tea/porridge with milk within 24 hours before the survey (in Kiswahili: Vinywaji vywenye maziwa) were statistically more likely to have stunting. Even though the question about feeding pattern was only for the 24 hours before the survey, such behavior could reflect daily routines in the household. According to observation of households in the study community, some caregivers were giving tea or porridge with milk to their children instead of a meal. As a result, some children did not have 3 meals a day, making them more vulnerable to stunting compared with those children who were not given tea or porridge as a meal. Some caregivers in households with severe food insecurity did not give such food to their children and those children were more likely to attain a nearly normal growth level. These caregivers can be a good model to optimize feeding practices with the locally available foodstuffs even in food insecure conditions. Further investigation in this matter is important to seek a community-level solution to prevent childhood stunting.

Children in the second and third year of life in the severely food insecure group were significantly more likely to have stunting compared with children 0 to 5 months old (Table 3). The following scenario can be assumed: up to 2 years old, a caregiver or mother gives breast milk mainly or as a complementary food to children. Actually, the proportion of breastfed children among our participants becomes zero by 30 months old from our survey data. As the children grow, the caregiver or mother stops giving breast milk and complementary food and shifts to improper feeding practices like providing tea or porridge with milk as a meal. Children then become chronically undernourished at this age. In this scenario, education focused on caregivers' feeding habits of complementary food for 2 to 3-year-old children can help prevent childhood stunting [27]. Further studies might be necessary to determine the right types of interventions for each community with the problems of childhood stunting and food insecurity.

The presence of jigger flea infection (tungiasis) might have an effect on child stunting in food insecure households, although in our study it was not significant. Tungiasis is a neglected ectoparasitic disease in resource-poor communities; however, the influence of this indigenous insect on younger children has not been thoroughly examined [28]. To date, only a few studies about the ecological description of jiggers have been conducted in Ethiopia [29], Cameroon [30], Brazil [31], and Nigeria [32]. Indeed, the majority of the children in this study, especially young children, did not wear shoes, which increases their risk of contracting jiggers. Other parasitic infections, like hookworm, which causes malnutrition and anemia, can simultaneously infect children in unhygienic conditions like this study area and contribute to stunting [33,34]. Further investigation on stunting and tungiasis, as well as load reduction of tungiasis, is necessary to help combat stunting [35].

In households in the non-severe food insecure group, animal rearing was significantly associated with childhood stunting. The presence of siblings of preschool age was not significant, but it was marginally associated. These results may indicate that childhood stunting is affected by caregivers who are less readily available for feeding children on a daily basis. The impact of caregivers' care for infants and young children has been widely acknowledged [36,37]. Some studies have also reported that limited household resources due to the presence of many children negatively influences their nutritional status [38-40]. Furthermore, since their illiterate elder siblings tend to remain in the house longer, caregivers who have many illiterate children may need to allocate psychological and material resources in the household for them. Therefore, last- or next-to-last-born children are less likely to have sufficient meals. In addition, caregivers may not be able to pay sufficient attention to children under 5 years old due to the need to attend to their own responsibilities. Thus, further long-term research about the conditions of intra-household food access, especially for families with illiterate children, is needed. A consensus regarding the importance of public education for children and family planning for parents is also required because caregivers play an important role in the development of healthy infants and young children. In addition, social support such as having assistants to help caregivers at the household level, is urgently required for adequate child growth [41].

In both groups, children of households in the highest SES category were less likely to have stunting. Some studies have identified socioeconomic inequality as a key factor in chronic childhood malnutrition [42,43]. According to the data from the HDSS in this area, the properties of homes used for calculation of SES by PCA are not very diverse in that a large majority of households had wood and mud walls (85.8%) and earth, dung, or sand floors (88.5%), with at least one plot of family land or family members who owned land (96.8%) [20]. Even though SES was divided into 4 categories by PCA, the range was narrow. This variable, therefore, can be interpreted as a controlling factor of SES to evaluate the relationship between childhood stunting and other factors.

There are several limitations in this study. Seasonal changes in the prevalence of stunted children in rural areas of developing countries have been reported [44,45]. Since this study is based on a cross-sectional design, any potential longitudinal relationships between stunted children and seasonal nutritional environmental changes were difficult to assess. Furthermore, the number of children in the study was not large enough to assess factors associated with stunting when we stratified by factors, e.g., food security level and age group. A larger number of children should be recruited to analyze for factor-stratified associations. Additionally, some feeding practices like giving tea/porridge with milk could not be evaluated adequately in this study. Not only increasing the number of subjects in the study, but also deepening the study contents, e.g., anthropological components, should be necessary.

6.5   CONCLUSIONS

A quarter of the children under 5 years old in the study area were found to suffer from chronic malnutrition. In the non-severe food insecurity group, animal rearing and SES were factors significantly associated with chronic malnutrition according to food insecurity level. The number of siblings of preschool age was not significantly associated, but was marginally associated. In the severely food insecure group, tea/porridge with milk and child age were significantly associated with child stunting. In other rural community settings of sub-Saharan Africa, the same situation could be happening. Our results suggest that countermeasures against childhood stunting should be optimized according to evidence observed in each community.

REFERENCES

1. Bhutta ZA, Das JK, Rizvi A, Gaffey MF, Walker N, Horton S, et al. Evidence-based interventions for improvement of maternal and child nutrition: what can be done and at what cost? Lancet. 2013;382(9890):452–77.

2. Black RE, Victora CG, Walker SP, Bhutta ZA, Christian P, de Onis M, et al. Maternal and child undernutrition and overweight in low-income and middle-income countries. Lancet. 2013;382(9890):427–51.

3. Victora CG, Adair L, Fall C, Hallal PC, Martorell R, Richter L, et al. Maternal and child undernutrition: consequences for adult health and human capital. Lancet. 2008;371(9609):340–57.

4. Shrimpton R, Victora CG, de Onis M, Lima RC, Blossner M, Clugston G. Worldwide timing of growth faltering: implications for nutritional interventions. Pediatrics. 2001;107(5):E75.

5. Dowdney L, Skuse D, Morris K, Pickles A. Short normal children and environmental disadvantage: a longitudinal study of growth and cognitive development from 4 to 11 years. J Child Psychol Psychiatr. 1998;39(7):1017–29.

6. World Health Organization. WHO child growth standards : length/height-for-age, weight-for-age, weight-for-length, weight-forheight and body mass index-for-age : methods and development. Geneva: WHO Press; 2006.

7. United Nations Children's Fund (UNICEF). Improving child nutrition: the achievable imperative for global progress. New York: United Nations Children's Fund; 2013.

8. Müller O, Krawinkel M. Malnutrition and health in developing countries. CMAJ. 2005;173(3):279–86.

9. Saleemi MA, Ashraf RN, Mellander L, Zaman S. Determinants of stunting at 6, 12, 24 and 60 months and postnatal linear growth in Pakistani children. Acta Paediatr. 2001;90(11):1304–8.

10. Rose-Jacobs R, Black MM, Casey PH, Cook JT, Cutts DB, Chilton M, et al. Household food insecurity: associations with at-risk infant and toddler development. Pediatrics. 2008;121(1):65–72.

11. Bhutta ZA, Ahmed T, Black RE, Cousens S, Dewey K, Giugliani E, et al. What works? Interventions for maternal and child undernutrition and survival. Lancet. 2008;371(9610):417–40.

12. Iwanaga Y, Tokunaga M, Ikuta S, Inatomi H, Araki M, Nakao Y, et al. Factors associated with nutritional status in children aged 6–24 months in Central African Republic: an anthropometric study at health centers in Bangui. J Int Health. 2009;24(4):289–98.

13. Kanjilal B, Mazumdar PG, Mukherjee M, Rahman MH. Nutritional status of children in India: household socio-economic condition as the contextual determinant. Int J Equity Health. 2010;9(1):19.

14. Abubakar A, Holding P, Mwangome M, Maitland K. Maternal perceptions of factors contributing to severe under-nutrition among children in a rural African setting. Rural Remote Health. 2011;11:1423.

15. Quisumbing AR. Male–female differences in agricultural productivity: methodological issues and empirical evidence. World Dev. 1996;24(10):1579–95.

16. Ayieko MA, Midikila KF. Seasonality of food supply, coping strategies and child nutritional outcome in Sabatia-Kenya. Adv J Food Sci Technol. 2010;2(5):279–85.

17. Hotta M, Li Y, Anme T, Ushijima H. Risk factors for low Kaup index among children in rural ethnic minority areas of Yunnan, China. Pediatr Int. 2005;47(2):147–53.

18. Van De Poel E, Hosseinpoor AR, Speybroeck N, Van Ourti T, Vega J. Socioeconomic inequality in malnutrition in developing countries. Bull World Health Organ. 2008;86(4):282–91.

19. Kenya National Bureau of Statistics (KNBS), ICF Macro. Kenya demographic and health survey 2008–2009. Calverton, Maryland: KNBS and ICF Macro; 2010.

20. Kaneko S, K'Opiyo J, Kiche I, Wanyua S, Goto K, Tanaka J, et al. Health and demographic surveillance system in the western and coastal areas of Kenya: an infrastructure for epidemiologic studies in Africa. J Epidemiol. 2012;22(3):276–85.

21. Swindale A, Bilinsky P. Development of a universally applicable household food insecurity measurement tool: process, current status, and outstanding issues. J Nutr. 2006;136(5):1449S–52.

22. Coates J, Swindale A, Bilinsky P. Household Food Insecurity Access Scale (HFIAS) for measurement of household food access: indicator guide. Washington, D.C: Food and Nutrition Technical Assistance Project, Academy for Educational Development; 2006.

23. Gwatkin DR, Rustein S, Johnson K, Pande RP, Wagstaff A. Socio-economic differences in health, nutrition, and population in Bangladesh. Washington, D.C: HNP/Poverty Thematic Group of The World Bank; 2000.

24. Saha KK, Frongillo EA, Alam DS, Arifeen SE, Persson LÅ, Rasmussen KM. Household food security is associated with growth of infants and young children in rural Bangladesh. Public Health Nutr. 2009;12(9):1556–62.

25. Ali D, Saha KK, Nguyen PH, Diressie MT, Ruel MT, Menon P, et al. Household food insecurity is associated with higher child undernutrition in Bangladesh, Ethiopia, and Vietnam, but the effect is not mediated by child dietary diversity. J Nutr. 2013; 143(12): 2015–21.

26. Remans R, Pronyk PM, Fanzo JC, Chen J, Palm CA, Nemser B, et al. Multisector intervention to accelerate reductions in child stunting: an observational study from 9 sub-Saharan African countries. Am J Clin Nutr. 2011;94(6):1632–42.

27. Imdad A, Yakoob MY, Bhutta ZA. Impact of maternal education about complementary feeding and provision of complementary foods on child growth in developing countries. BMC Public Health. 2011;11 Suppl 3:S25.

28. Heukelbach J, Sales De Oliveira FA, Hesse G, Feldmeier H. Tungiasis: a neglected health problem of poor communities. Trop Med Int Health. 2001;6(4):267–72.

29. Hall A, Kassa T, Demissie T, Degefie T, Lee S. National survey of the health and nutrition of schoolchildren in Ethiopia. Trop Med Int Health. 2008;13(12):1518–26.

30. Collins G, McLeod T, Konfor NI, Lamnyam CB, Ngarka L, Njamnshi NL. Tungiasis: a neglected health problem in rural Cameroon. Int J Collaborative Res Intern Med Public Health. 2009;1(1):2–10.

31. Heukelbach J, Wilcke T, Eisele M, Feldmeier H. Ectopic localization of tungiasis. Am J Trop Med Hyg. 2002;67(2 SUPPL):214–6.

32. Ugbomoiko US, Ariza L, Ofoezie IE, Heukelbach J. Risk factors for tungiasis in Nigeria: identification of targets for effective intervention. PLoS Negl Trop Dis. 2007;1(3):e87.

33. Feldmeier H, Sentongo E, Krantz I. Tungiasis (sand flea disease): a parasitic disease with particular challenges for public health. Eur J Clin Microbiol Infect Dis. 2013;32(1):19–26.

34. Feldmeier H, Heukelbach J. Epidermal parasitic skin diseases: a neglected category of poverty-associated plagues. Bull World Health Organ. 2009;87(2):152–9.

35. Pilger D, Schwalfenberg S, Heukelbach J, Witt L, Mencke N, Khakban A, et al. Controlling tungiasis in an impoverished community: an intervention study. PLoS Negl Trop Dis. 2008; 2(10), e324.

36. Stansbury JP, Leonard WR, Dewalt KM. Caretakers, child care practices, and growth failure in Highland Ecuador. Med Anthropol Q. 2000;14(2):224–41.

37. Tunçbilek E, Ünalan T, Coşkun T. Indicators of nutritional status in Turkish preschool children: Results of Turkish Demographic and Health Survey 1993. J Trop Pediatr. 1996;42(2):78–84.

38. Vitolo MR, Gama CM, Bortolini GA, Campagnolo PDB, Drachler MDL. Some risk factors associated with overweight, stunting and wasting among children under 5 years old. J Pediatr (Rio J). 2008;84(3):251–7.

39. Victora CG, Vaughan JP, Kirkwood BR, Martines JC, Barcelos LB. Risk factors for malnutrition in Brazilian children: the role of social and environmental variables. Bull World Health Organ. 1986;64(2):299–309.

40. Bronte-Tinkew J, Dejong G. Children's nutrition in Jamaica: do household structure and household economic resources matter? Soc Sci Med. 2004;58(3):499–514.

41. Bégin F, Frongillo Jr EA, Delisle H. Caregiver behaviors and resources influence child height-for-age in rural Chad. J Nutr. 1999;129(3):680–6.

42. Hong R. Effect of economic inequality on chronic childhood undernutrition in Ghana. Public Health Nutr. 2007;10(4):371–8.

43. Menon P, Ruel MT, Morris SS. Socio-economic differentials in child stunting are consistently larger in urban than in rural areas. Food Nutr Bull. 2000;21(3):282–9.

44. Brown KH, Black RE, Becker S. Seasonal changes in nutritional status and the prevalence of malnutrition in a longitudinal study of young children in rural Bangladesh. Am J Clin Nutr. 1982;36(2):303–13.

45. Kigutha HN, Van Staveren WA, Veerman W, Hautvast JGAJ. Child malnutrition in poor smallholder households in rural Kenya: an in-depth situation analysis. Eur J Clin Nutr. 1995;49(9):691–702.

PART III

Food Security and Mental and Physical Health

CHAPTER 7

Beyond Nutrition: Hunger and Its Impact on the Health of Young Canadians

William Pickett, Valerie Michaelson, and Colleen Davison

7.1 INTRODUCTION

Consistent access to a healthy food supply is an important determinant of health and a fundamental human right (World Food Programme 2007). In children, food is required to nurture healthy growth and development but is related to the vitality of the whole person, including their emotional and social well-being (World Food Programme 2007). During the adolescent years, the need for intake of sufficient calories and essential nutrients increases (Dwyer 1993) and food insufficiencies can lead to ongoing health problems (Molcho et al. 2007).

Hunger during childhood is related to poor food and nutritional environments in families (Robaina and Martin 2013; Alaimo et al. 2001). It is also prognostic for negative child health outcomes such as obesity (Nackers and Appelhans 2013), poor self-rated health (Niclasen et al. 2013a, b), increased physical symptoms and associated medicine use (Niclasen et al. 2013a, b), poorer emotional health (Melchior et al. 2012), lower health-related quality of life (Casey et al. 2005), and impaired physical function (Casey et al. 2005). Hunger associated with poor nutrition also makes children vulnerable to disease due to infections (World Food Programme 2007). Manifestations of hunger are sometimes overt, but are often invisible, and reflect the powerlessness and vulnerability of those who suffer from its consequences (World Food Programme 2007).

Hunger caused by an inadequate or inconsistent food supply at home is part of a larger societal issue that is variably referred to as "food insecurity", "food poverty", or "food insufficiency" (Food and Agriculture Organization of the United Nations 1996). These terms refer to a myriad of situations where consistent physical and economic access to sufficient, safe and nutritious food of a person's preference cannot be assured (Food and Agriculture Organization of the United Nations 1996). This field of study is, however, challenging in that there are many different disciplines that are interested and there are subtle differences in the way that these concepts are approached. For example, a recent review suggests that in excess of 200 definitions exist for the term "food insecurity" alone (Food and Agricultural Organization of the United Nations 2013), making comparisons across studies and disciplines daunting.

Further, while the origins and health consequences of hunger have been studied extensively in adults (Stuff et al. 2004; Vozoris and Tarasuk 2003), few analogous large-scale studies exist for adolescents, and almost none in first world countries such as Canada. The etiology of hunger is tied to many obvious social factors including poverty (James et al. 1997) and the strength and organization of families and community networks (Fulkerson et al. 2006). Less evidence exists about the consequences of persistent hunger on the health and well-being of young people. The extent to which organized food and nutrition programs impact upon the long-term effects of hunger is also under-studied (Gelli and Daryanani 2013). Collectively, these represent important gaps in knowledge.

Our Canadian research group is involved in the Health Behavior in School-aged Children (HBSC) study. HBSC is a World Health Organization collaborative study of health and health risk behaviors. We performed a national study of hunger in populations of young people. We explored: (1) the prevalence of self-reported hunger and variations in reported hunger among groups of adolescents; (2) relations between hunger and several physical, emotional and social health outcomes, and; (3) whether such relations can be explained in part by socio-economic, family, and school-based contextual influences. Our aim was to provide foundational information to support the development of evidence-based prevention strategies, and we believe that this was achieved.

7.2   METHODS

7.2.1   Study Population and Procedures

HBSC involves written health surveys conducted in classroom settings, with a focus on the adolescent years (ages 11–15). It is administered every 4 years following a common international protocol (Freeman et al. 2011).

The 2009–2010 (cycle 6) Canadian sample was developed using a multistage, clustered strategy. The primary sampling unit was schools. All students within selected classrooms within those schools were approached to participate. The sample was stratified first by province/territory, then: type of school board (public vs. separate), urban–rural geographic status, school population size, and language of instruction (French vs. English). If a school board or school refused participation, a neighboring school board or school with similar characteristics was approached to participate. Standardized population weights were generated to account for oversampling and stratification criteria. Children from private schools, home schools, First Nations or Inuit reserves, street youth, incarcerated youth, and youth not providing informed consent (explicit or implicit, as per school board customs) were excluded. Response rates were 11/13 (84.6 %) at the province/territorial level (New Brunswick and Prince Edward Island were excluded), 436/765 (57.0 %) at the level of schools (404 of whom answered an administrators' questionnaire), and 26,078/33,868 (77.0 %) at the student level, with a weighted sample of 25,912 providing responses to a question on hunger.

The study protocol was approved by the Queen's University General Research Ethics Board. Written parental consent or implied (passive) consent was obtained, according to local school board customs.

7.2.2   Measures

7.2.2.1   Hunger

Students' perceptions of hunger were measured: "Some young people go to school or to bed hungry because there is not enough food at home. How often does this happen to you?" with response options of never, sometimes, often, or always. This item was piloted in six HBSC countries (Canada, Macedonia, Norway, Poland, Scotland, Wales) in the year 2000. Findings indicated that young people were interpreting the words of the question as a measure of social deprivation (Griebler et al. 2009). It has been used as an indicator of child hunger, and as well as a proxy indicator of socio-economic status and food availability. With respect to concurrent validity, reports from this hunger measure have been related to the many adverse health behaviors and outcomes (Riches 1997; Molcho et al. 2007; Mullen et al. 2002). It is not, however, possible to relate individual child reports of hunger to other "gold standard" measures.

7.2.2.2 Individual Health Outcomes

Adiposity Youth self-reported weight and height in metric or imperial units and body mass index (BMI) was calculated. To account for growth and maturation, children's BMI values were converted to age-and sex-specific levels and categorized into normal weight, overweight, or obese using standard international cut-points (Cole 1979).

Physical inactivity Moderate to vigorous physical activity was measured by taking an average of the responses to: "Over the past 7 days, on how many days were you physically active for a total of at least 60 min per day?" and "Over a typical or usual week, on how many days are you physically active for a total of at least 60 min per day?" (Prochaska et al. 2001). Physical inactivity was defined as a score of <4 days per week, aligned with the Canadian child physical activity guidelines (Nichol et al. 2009).

Frequent physical fighting Reports of two or more physical fights in the past 12 months were used to identify more young people who engaged in violence more frequently. Frequent physical fighting is a validated construct with extensive use in adolescent health surveys (Pickett et al. 2013; Brener et al. 1999).

Engagement in bullying and being a victim of bullying were assessed using items adapted from Olweus, and defined as perpetrating or being victimized by bullying while at school regularly (2 or 3 times per month to several times per week), following existing precedents (Kyriakides et al. 2006).

Frequency of talking back to teachers (4–6 vs. 1–3 on a 6-point scale where 1 was definitely not like me and 6 were definitely like me) was used as a measure of social delinquency.

7.2.2.3 Composite Health Outcomes

Psychosomatic symptoms Youth reported the frequency (5-point Likert-like scale ranging from rarely or never to almost every day) of the following psychosomatic symptoms: headache, stomach ache, backache, feeling low (depressed), irritability or bad temper, nervousness, difficulty in getting sleep, dizziness. These were combined into a composite scale with strong psychometric properties (Hetland et al. 2002). We later divided scores into categories, with the top category representing frequent (on average "weekly" or "daily") reporting of symptoms.

Emotional health scales Four existing composite scales were used to describe negative and then positive aspects of emotional health that involved different internalizing and externalizing behaviors (Freeman et al. 2011). These were conceptualized as follows: internalizing-negative (emotional problems); externalizing-negative (behavioral problems); internalizing-positive (emotional well-being), and externalizing-positive (pro-social behaviors).

7.2.2.4   Demographic Factors

Variables considered as descriptive covariates included: gender (boys vs. girls); school grade (6–8 vs. 9–10); immigration status (born in Canada, immigrated >5 years ago, immigrated within 1–5 years); family structure in the primary home (mother and father, mother and step-father, father and step-mother, mother only, father only, other); (all level 1), and geographic size of the residential community [rural (<1000 persons); small (1000–19,999 persons); medium (20,000–99,999 person); and large (≥100,000 persons) (level 2)].

7.2.2.5   Family and School Factors

Socio-economic status (level 1) Family affluence (FAS; a validated measure of socio-economic status) (Currie et al. 2008) was measured by assessing participants' answers to four items describing the material conditions of their household (respondents' own household bedrooms, family holidays, family vehicle ownership, family computer ownership). Responses to the items are summed on a nine-point scale with set cut-points for low (0–3), medium (4–5) and high (6–9) affluence.

Family characteristics (level 1) Each participant was asked "on average, how many times per week does your family sit down at the table together for dinner/supper?" (response options: zero through seven times) (Elgar et al. 2013). They were also asked "how often do you usually have breakfast (more than a glass of milk or fruit juice) on weekdays?" (response options: never through 5 days)

(Tarasuk and Vogt 2009). Participants were also asked about communication in the home, i.e., "How easy is it for you to talk to the following persons (categories included mother, father) about things that really bother you? "(5 response options: "very easy", "easy", "difficult", "very difficult", "don't have or see this person")" (Elgar et al. 2013).

School food and nutrition programs (level 2) The HBSC administrator's questionnaire contained items describing food and nutrition. Three internally consistent scales (Cronbach's alpha ranged from 0.77 to 0.91) described availability of healthy food choices available at school. Additional school items asked about access to nutritious food regardless of ability to pay; literacy programs related to healthy eating, breakfast and lunch programs, and specific educational opportunities aimed at nutrition (cooking classes, gardening classes, and field trips to grocery stores, farms or farmers markets).

7.2.3   Statistical Analysis

Data analyses were conducted with SAS 9.3 (SAS Institute, Cary, NC, 2010). Descriptive analyses were used to characterize the prevalence of hunger as perceived by students in the overall population, and then within-population subgroups. We also described socio-economic contexts, family characteristics and practices, and the presence of school food and nutrition programs in participating schools and then their relations with hunger.

We used a hierarchical approach to our modeling. The first step was the development of empty models for each of the 11 health outcomes. These partitioned the variance in each of the health outcomes attributable to level 1 (students) nested within level 2 (school) factors.

Next, bivariate logistic regression analyses were then conducted to model each of the 11 health outcomes described above (yes vs. no) as dependent variables, with reports of hunger as the independent variable. These models too accounted for the nested and clustered nature of the sampling scheme using the SAS PROC GLIMMIX procedure and by specifying the schools as random effects. We specified fixed betas but random intercepts after testing the fit of models that were based upon different assumptions. Standardized weights were also applied to account for variations in sampling between provinces and territories.

Next, a series of three separate adjusted logistic regression models that employed the same hierarchical approach were developed to explore the idea that relations between hunger and health could be explained by various factors: (1) family socio-economic conditions (Model 1; with family affluence treated as a level 1 variable); (2) family characteristics and practices (Model 2; with these treated as level 1 variables), and, (3) school food and nutrition programs (Model 3; with these treated as level 2 variables). For ease of interpretation, we adjusted for a standard set of Level 1 confounders in each of the three models (age, grade level, immigration status, and family structure of the primary home), with the latter two models also adjusted for family affluence. Model 1 and Model 2 therefore included only level 1 predictors but included school as a random effect to adjust for clustering. Model 3 included both level 1 and level 2 factors and school as a random effect. When interpreting the findings of the three models, substantial changes ($\geq 10\%$) in estimates towards the null for adjusted versus bivariate models were interpreted as evidence in support of the three separate explanations for the occurrence of hunger.

7.3   RESULTS

Overall, a weighted sample of 25,912 young people was included. Approximately 25 % of this sample reported going to school or bed hungry because there was not enough food at home at least "sometimes", with 3.8 % indicating that this occurred "often" or "always" (Table 1). No substantial variations in these proportions were observed by gender, grade level, immigration status, or community size.

TABLE 7.1   Hunger reported by young people in Canada: Canadian HBSC Study, 2010

Sub-group	Sample (n)	Percent (%) reporting going to school or bed hungry because there is not enough food at home			
		Never	Sometimes	Often	Always
Sample	25,912	74.9	21.4	2.8	1.0
By gender					
Boys	12,708	74.1	22.0	2.8	1.1
Girls	13,198	75.6	20.8	2.7	0.9
By grade level					
6–8	15,523	73.6	22.8	2.7	0.9
9–10	10.388	76.8	19.2	2.8	1.2
By immigration status					
Born in Canada	13,951	75.9	20.5	2.6	0.9
Immigrant: recent	1199	72.7	22.9	2.8	1.6
Immigrant: not recent	6.097	72.0	23.9	3.0	1.1

TABLE 7.1   *(Continued)*

Sub-group	Sample (n)	Percent (%) reporting going to school or bed hungry because there is not enough food at home			
		Never	Sometimes	Often	Always
By family structure of primary home					
Both parents	16,890	77.0	19.9	2.2	0.9
Mother and step-father	1961	72.1	23.7	3.2	1.0
Father and step-mother	506	77.3	19.4	3.0	0.9
Mother only	3805	70.9	24.1	3.9	1.1
Father only	814	65.8	27.6	4.8	1.7
Other	1177	69.0	25.7	3.8	1.4
By geographic center size					
Rural or remote	977	77.4	19.6	1.9	1.1
Small	10,712	75.4	21.3	2.5	0.9
Medium	5688	75.2	21.0	2.8	1.0
Large	8538	74.4	21.4	3.0	1.2

Hunger related to a number of socio-economic and family factors, and we present some illustrative examples here. More frequent levels of hunger were reported when respondents came from single parent and "other" versus two parent family structures (Table 1). The prevalence of hunger declined with higher reported levels of family affluence (Fig. 1). Strong and consistent declines in hunger were also observed with increased participation in family meals (Fig. 2).

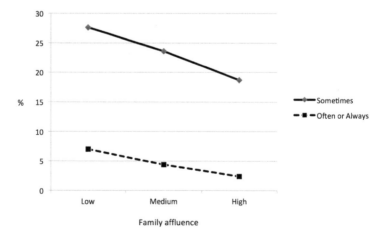

FIGURE 7.1   Percentage of young people reporting hunger by level of family affluence: Canadian HBSC Study, 2010

Similar associations were evident between improved levels of family communication and reduced experiences of hunger, and increased breakfast eating and reduced hunger.

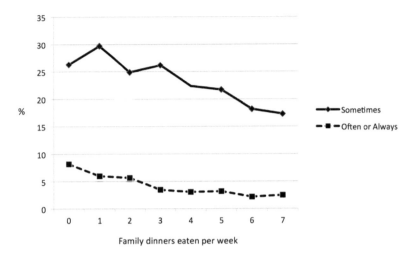

FIGURE 7.2   Percentage of young people reporting hunger by number of family dinners eaten together per week at home: Canadian HBSC Study, 2010

Substantial proportions of Canadian schools are involved in formal efforts to address hunger, food and the nutritional needs of children (Table 2). Formal school programs were aimed at nutritional education, healthy eating, as well as the provision of food at a reasonable cost. However, reported levels of "going to school or bed hungry" were not associated with these school programs in a consistent or strong manner (Fig. 3).

TABLE 7.2   Food environments reported by school administrators in Canada: Canadian HBSC Study, 2010

Variable	% Yes
Cafeteria food and nutrition programs ($n = 396$ responding schools)	
Healthy food choices at a reasonable or subsidized price	46.5
Healthy eating promotional materials	41.9
Daily healthy eating specials	38.6
Healthy eating program (e.g., eat smart or independent program)	34.3
Other initiative to promote healthy eating	6.6

TABLE 7.2 *(Continued)*

Variable	% Yes
Snack bar food and nutrition programs (*n* = 396 responding schools)	
Healthy food choices at a reasonable or subsidized price	20.5
Healthy eating promotional materials	13.4
Daily healthy eating specials	6.8
Healthy eating program (e.g., eat smart or independent program)	5.6
Other initiative to promote healthy eating	2.5
Vending machine food and nutrition programs (*n* = 396 responding schools)	
Healthy food choices at a reasonable or subsidized price	23.2
Healthy eating promotional materials	6.1
Daily healthy eating specials	2.0
Healthy eating program (e.g., eat smart or independent program)	2.5
Other initiative to promote healthy eating	0.8
Other food and nutrition initiatives (number of responding schools varies)	
All students, regardless of ability to pay, have access to fruits and vegetables (*n* = 396)	
At least sometimes during year	67.3
Entire year	39.9
Occasional or seasonal	27.3
Media literacy related to healthy eating (*n* = 404)	67.3
Healthy food choices during lunch program (*n* = 391)	66.8
Healthy food choices during breakfast program (*n* = 387)	57.9
Cooking classes (*n* = 404)	58.9
Field trips to local grocery stores (*n* = 404)	35.6
Field trips to farms or farmers markets (*n* = 404)	26.5
Gardening classes (growing produce) (*n* = 404)	15.3

Relations between the self-reported level of hunger and health outcomes are summarized below and in Table 3. The percentage of variance that was observed at the school level varied from 0.9 to 10.3 %, justifying the use of a multi-level or hierarchical modeling approach. Results indicated by the bivariate models were remarkably consistent. Each showed statistically significant increases in risk for all negative individual and composite health outcomes studied, and similar decreases in risk for the two positive individual health outcomes. Adjusted Model 1 shows that relations between hunger and health remained basically unchanged when we controlled for our level 1 measure of self-reported family affluence. Adjusted Model 2 indicated consistent changes in the odds ratio estimates towards the null for all 11 outcomes once the level 1 family variables were controlled for. These included measures of frequency of engagement in family dinners, breakfasts eaten by young people during the school week, and ease of communication with mothers and fathers. Adjusted Model 3 shows that the odds ratio estimates remained relatively unchanged from the bivariate estimates following adjustment for level 2 indicators of school food and nutrition programs. The latter included summary scales describing food availability at school, and individual measures describing access to food at school regardless of ability to pay, breakfast and lunch programs, and classes that focused on diet and nutrition.

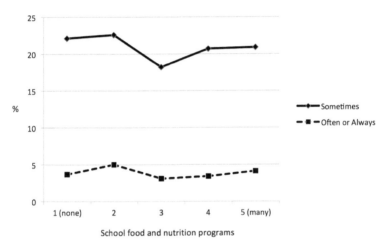

FIGURE 7.3   Percentage of young people reporting hunger by reported levels of school food and nutrition programs in school cafeterias: Canadian HBSC Study, 2010.

7.4   DISCUSSION

This national study demonstrated that hunger was common among young Canadians. It confirmed the presence of relations between hunger and poverty, but perhaps less predictably, showed that hunger is also related to a number of common family characteristics including their structure, communication patterns, and meal practices, irrespective of socio-economic status. We also confirmed the existence of strong relations between going to school or bed hungry and a large number of negative health outcomes. And finally, we showed that

TABLE 7.3 Relationships between hunger and individual and composite physical, emotional and social health outcomes: Canadian HBSC Study, 2010

Health outcome: level of food insecurity	% with Health outcome	OR (95 % CI)[d]			
		Bivariate Models	Adjusted Model 1: family socio-economic[a]	Adjusted Model 2: family characteristics and practices[b]	Adjusted Model 3: school food and nutrition programs[c]
Individual health outcomes					
Overweight/obese					
Never	20.0	1.00	1.00	1.00	1.00
Sometimes	24.4	1.28 (1.18–1.39)	1.26 (1.16–1.37)	1.25 (1.14–1.36)	1.25 (1.14–1.37)
Often or always	24.9	1.33 (1.11–1.58)	1.23 (1.01–1.48)	1.14 (0.94–1.39)	1.28 (1.05–1.56)
Physically inactive					
Never	33.4	1.00	1.00	1.00	1.00
Sometimes	39.7	1.28 (1.20–1.37)	1.24 (1.16–1.33)	1.15 (1.06–1.23)	1.23 (1.14–1.32)
Often or always	44.8	1.53 (1.34–1.76)	1.44 (1.24–1.67)	1.31 (1.12–1.53)	1.41 (1.20–1.60)
Frequent physical fighting					
Never	17.9	1.00	1.00	1.00	1.00
Sometimes	22.7	1.36 (1.26–1.46)	1.32 (1.21–1.43)	1.18 (1.08–1.29)	1.30 (1.19–1.42)
Often or always	26.5	1.66 (1.42–1.94)	1.76 (1.48–2.09)	1.42 (1.19–1.70)	1.81 (1.51–2.16)
Frequent bullying					
Never	14.7	1.00	1.00	1.00	1.00
Sometimes	18.9	1.33 (1.23–1.45)	1.31 (1.20–1.42)	1.15 (1.05–1.26)	1.31 (1.20–1.44)
Often or always	29.0	2.33 (2.00–2.70)	2.31 (1.96–2.72)	1.76 (1.48–2.09)	2.31 (1.95–2.74)

TABLE 7.3 (*Continued*)

Health outcome: level of food insecurity	% with Health outcome	OR (95 % CI)[d]			
		Bivariate Models	Adjusted Model 1: family socio-economic[a]	Adjusted Model 2: family characteristics and practices[b]	Adjusted Model 3: school food and nutrition programs[c]
Frequent victimization by bullying					
Never	26.0	1.00	1.00	1.00	1.00
Sometimes	38.5	1.80 (1.68–1.92)	1.76 (1.66–1.89)	1.62 (1.51–1.75)	1.81 (1.69–1.95)
Often or always	48.0	2.74 (2.39–3.13)	2.53 (2.19–2.93)	2.06 (1.77–2.40)	2.61 (2.24–3.04)
Talk back to teachers					
Never	17.8	1.00	1.00	1.00	1.00
Sometimes	23.4	1.34 (1.24–1.46)	1.33 (1.22–1.45)	1.25 (1.14–1.37)	1.31 (1.20–1.44)
Often or always	30.6	1.93 (1.63–2.27)	1.73 (1.45–2.06)	1.50 (1.25–1.81)	1.78 (1.48–2.15)
Composite health outcomes					
Frequent psychosomatic symptoms					
Never	24.1	1.00	1.00	1.00	1.00
Sometimes	35.4	1.78 (1.66–1.90)	1.84 (1.71–1.99)	1.56 (1.44–1.69)	1.88 (1.74–2.04)
Often or always	55.1	3.85 (3.35–4.43)	4.27 (3.65–4.98)	3.24 (2.74–3.84)	4.42 (3.75–5.21)
Internalizing problems					
Never	29.0	1.00	1.00	1.00	1.00
Sometimes	45.7	2.09 (1.97–2.23)	2.15 (2.01–2.30)	1.89 (1.76–2.03)	2.12 (1.97–2.27)
Often or always	60.4	3.78 (3.30–4.33)	3.82 (3.29–4.44)	2.96 (2.52–3.48)	3.78 (3.23–4.42)

TABLE 7.3 (*Continued*)

Health outcome: level of food insecurity	% with Health outcome	OR (95 % CI)[d]			
		Bivariate Models	Adjusted Model 1: family socio-economic[a]	Adjusted Model 2: family characteristics and practices[b]	Adjusted Model 3: school food and nutrition programs[c]
Externalizing problems					
Never	33.8	1.00	1.00	1.00	1.00
Sometimes	39.9	1.28 (1.19–1.36)	1.24 (1.15–1.33)	1.11 (1.03–1.19)	1.21 (1.12–1.30)
Often or always	52.4	2.02 (1.75–2.33)	2.00 (1.72–2.32)	1.59 (1.36–1.86)	2.05 (1.75–2.40)
Emotional well-being					
Never	40.0	1.00	1.00	1.00	1.00
Sometimes	28.5	0.56 (0.53–0.60)	0.56 (0.52–0.61)	0.67 (0.62–0.73)	0.58 (0.53–0.62)
Often or always	22.5	0.42 (0.36–0.49)	0.45 (0.38–0.54)	0.55 (0.45–0.67)	0.44 (0.36–0.53)
Pro-social behavior					
Never	32.6	1.00	1.00	1.00	1.00
Sometimes	28.2	0.81 (0.75–0.86)	0.82 (0.77–0.88)	0.89 (0.83–0.96)	0.84 (0.78–0.90)
Often or always	29.0	0.85 (0.73–0.99)	0.83 (0.71–0.98)	0.88 (0.74–1.04)	0.85 (0.72–1.01)

[a] Adjusted Model 1. Adjusted for level 1 variables of age, gender, immigration status, family structure, and family affluence
[b] Adjusted Model 2. Adjusted for level 1 variables of age, gender, immigration status, family structure, family affluence, communication with father, communication with mother, family dinners, frequency of breakfast consumption
[c] Adjusted Model 3. Adjusted for level 1 variables of age, gender, immigration status, family structure, family affluence, and level 2 variables of school breakfast and lunch programs, availability of food at cost, cooking classes, gardening classes, school cafeteria programs, school snack bar programs
[d] All models also include school as a random effect to account for clustering

while these latter relations were in part accounted for by family characteristics, there was no evidence of similar mediation effects by our measures of socio-economic status or our assessment of school-based food and nutrition programs.

Basic information on the prevalence of hunger is informative. In a developed country such as Canada, it is remarkable that up to 25 % of young people report going to school or bed hungry due to a lack of food in the home at least occasionally, with 4 % reporting this often or always. Even considering the opportunity for misclassification, these estimates are sobering. By extrapolation and using population counts from the 2011 Census of Population (Statistics Canada 2014), the 3.8 % figure translates into a total of 73,000 Canadian children aged 11–15 years reporting going to school or bed hungry as indicated by our measure (54,000 "often", 19,000 "always"). Reported prevalence levels are consistent with historical reports for child populations (Tarasuk and Vogt 2009), and they point to a quiet public health problem in a wealthy country that shows that hunger is not just experienced in economically disadvantaged nations.

We also confirmed a number of gradients consistent with the idea that hunger has social origins. We and others (Molcho et al. 2007) have shown that hunger due to having insufficient food at home occurs not only in disadvantaged families, but in affluent families as well. In addition, our analyses did not find expected relations between school-based food and nutrition programs and going to school or bed hungry. While this was somewhat expected because the wording of the question specified hunger in non-school hours, it does point to possible limitations of school programs for experiences of overall hunger, and may suggest a more distal role of schools in this etiological pathway. This is not to say that programs that provide food to children are not of value. Rather, it suggests that hunger is a more ubiquitous problem, and while concentrated within impoverished families and a spectrum of schools who serve socio-economically disadvantaged populations, it is not unique to them. Hunger crosses cultures and populations, and feeding the hungry in all parts of society should always remain a priority (US Department of Agriculture 2013; Melbye et al. 2013).

Going to school or bed hungry was also remarkably consistent in its associations with negative health outcomes. It is telling that these relations persisted when we controlled for our available measure of socio-economic status. This suggests that poverty alone is less likely to explain why hunger results in various states of impaired health. Other social explanations are warranted. Next, when we controlled for school-based food and nutrition programs, the observed negative health relations persisted. While such programs address an obvious need, they do not eliminate the persistent negative health effects of a home without adequate organization or resources to ensure a consistent and adequate food supply. While addressing child hunger directly with food and nutrition programs is an essential moral and social responsibility, it is only part of the solution to a more complex social problem.

Negative health outcomes related to hunger may be caused not only by lack of food, but by more insidious feelings caused by food insecurity at home. Relations between hunger and the various health effects were attenuated, and perhaps partially mediated, when home-based factors were controlled for in our models. Speculatively, much of the challenge in addressing this hunger problem lies with addressing social factors that originate in the home. The latter may include things such as the stress that comes with having limited or sporadic access to food as well as feelings of a lack of control in life, injustice, questioning of one's self worth, stress around problems of food access, and associated alienation (Coates et al. 2006).

A more holistic approach has been proposed to address the negative effects of hunger on adolescents, with a focus on the concept of "care" (Longhurst and Tomkins 1995). The UN declaration of the rights of the child echoes this basic holistic need (United Nations 1959). Beyond the right to adequate nutrition, a focus on care recognizes that for optimal development, children need love and understanding as well as "an atmosphere of affection and of moral and material security" (United Nations 1959). The role of care in terms of affection, emotional support, and effective allocation of resources within an atmosphere of stability and security has a direct influence on child nutritional outcomes (Engle et al. 2000; Engle and Lida 1999). Even in situations of poverty where there is household food insecurity and children are exposed to unhealthy physical and social environments, providing enhanced care can improve nutritional outcomes (Longhurst and Tomkins 1995).

In the 1990s, care was introduced as a fundamental component of nutritional well-being in young children (Engle et al. 2000; United Nations Children's Fund 1990). Care has more recently been understood as the behaviors and practices by caregivers to provide the food, health care, stimulation and emotional support that are needed for optimal child health and development (Engle et al. 2000). Ensuring adequate care also involves provision of the time, attention and support required to meet a range of needs in the developing child (physical, mental, emotional and social) (Longhurst and Tomkins 1995). This suggests the need for an integrative approach to the mediation of the consistent negative effects of hunger in children. A holistic approach would certainly include the provision of food, but would also look at the family context and the basic essential elements of care that children require.

If the problem of food insecurity is in the home, innovative solutions to help families are needed there, and not just in community settings. Providing food is one simple—though essential—solution. The root of the issue—the essential human issue—is much more complex. It is connected to our value as human beings and to equity and well-being; not just in filling empty stomachs. In a developed country of such wealth and relative peace, the existence of hunger among children in Canada is a moral failing on the part of society. For the good of all, addressing all aspects of this complex issue needs to become an essential priority, not only by government, but by community leaders, educators, and all capable adults.

Strengths of our study include the size of the study population and its national scope. The analysis was novel and addressed several practical questions about hunger, its distribution within adolescent society, its possible health consequences, and potential explanations. Limitations include the cross-sectional HBSC design, which is not as ideal as longitudinal designs for causal inference. Our use of a single item to measure a very complex construct will result in some misclassification. It is certainly possible that food is available in homes, and children report going to school or bed hungry because they do not like the selection of food available, or do not wish to prepare it for consumption. A strength of this child measure is that it is based upon a simple question that is asked directly to children. This might be less likely to be subject to parental reporting biases. We also had no information on adult factors that could contribute to family dysfunction (e.g., violence, mental health) and then hunger. Finally, the HBSC sampling strategy excluded some adolescent groups that may be at higher risk for hunger (e.g., youth on reserves and street youth), which may impact upon the external validity of our findings.

7.5 CONCLUSION

In this national study of adolescent Canadians, we document the prevalence of going to school or bed hungry due to having insufficient food at home. This type of hunger was related to a number of negative emotional, physical and social health outcomes. Such relations are modified by family practices, but less so by socio-economic factors or school-based food and nutrition programs. Future research, both quantitative and qualitative, is required to understand fully the social circumstances that result in adolescent hunger. Our findings also point to a need for a focus on practical family measures to truly ameliorate the root causes of this problem and its immediate consequences in terms of child health. While food programs are one important component of addressing hunger in Canadian children, we suggest that a more integrative approach with a focus on care is needed.

REFERENCES

1. Alaimo K, Olson CM, Frongillo EA (2001) Low family income and food insufficiency in relation to overweight in children: is there a paradox? Arch Ped Adolesc Med 155:1161–1167
2. Brener ND, Simon TR, Krug EG, Lowry R (1999) Recent trends in violence-related behaviours among high school students in the United States. JAMA 282(5):440–446
3. Casey PH, Szeto KL, Robbins JM et al (2005) Child health-related quality of life and household food security. Arch Pediatr Adolesc Med 159(1):51–56
4. Coates J, Frongillo EA, Rogers BL, Webb P, Wilde PE, Houser R (2006) Commonalities in the experience of household food insecurity across cultures: what are measures missing? J Nutr 136:1438S–1448S
5. Cole TJ (1979) A method for assessing age-standardized weight-for-height in children seen cross-sectionally. Ann Hum Biol 6:249–268
6. Currie C, Molcho M, Boyce W, Holstein B, Torsheim T, Richter M (2008) Researching health inequalities in adolescents: the development of the Health Behaviour in School-Aged Children (HBSC) family affluence scale. Soc Sci Med 66(6):1429–1436
7. Currie C, Nic Gabhainn S, Godeau E, International HBSC Network Coordinating Committee (2009) The Health Behaviour in School-aged Children: WHO Collaborative Cross National (HBSC) study: origins, concept, history and development 1982–2008. Int J Public Health 54(2):131–139
8. Dwyer JT (1993) Childhood, youth and old age. In: Garrow JS, James WPT (eds) Human nutrition and dietetics. Churchill-Livingstone, Edinburgh, pp 394–408
9. Elgar RJ, Craig W, Trites SJ (2013) Family dinners, communication, and mental health in Canadian adolescents. J Adolesc Health 52(4):433–438
10. Engle PL, Lida L (1999) The role of care in programmatic actions for nutrition: designing programmes involving care. Food Nutr Bull 20(1):121–135
11. Engle PL, Bentley M, Pelto G (2000) The role of care in nutrition programmes: current research and a research agenda. Proc Nutr Soc 59:25–35
12. Food and Agricultural Organization of the United Nations (2013) Commodity policy and projections service, commodities and trade division. Trade reforms and food security: conceptualizing the linkages. ftp://ftp.fao.org/docrep/fao/005/y4671e/y4671e00.pdf. Accessed 1 April 2014
13. Food and Agriculture Organization of the United Nations (1996) Rome Declaration on World Food Security and World Food Summit Plan of Action. http://www.fao.org/docrep/003/w3613e/w3613e00.htm. Accessed 1 Jan 2013
14. Food and Nutrition Service, US Department of Agriculture (2013) National School Lunch Program and School Breakfast Program: nutrition standards for all foods sold in school

as required by the Healthy, Hunger-Free Kids Act of 2010. Interim final rule. Fed Regist 78(125):39067–39120

15. Freeman JG, King M, Pickett W et al (2011) The health of Canada's young people: a mental health focus. Public Health Agency of Canada, Ottawa. Cat. no.: hP15-13/2011E-PDF, ISBN: hP15-13/2011E, 194p

16. Fulkerson JA, Story M, Mellin A, Leffert N, Neumark-Sztainer D, French FA (2006) Family dinner meal frequency and adolescent development: relationships with developmental assets and high-risk behaviors. J Adolesc Health 39:337e45

17. Gelli A, Daryanani R (2013) Are school feeding programs in low-income settings sustainable? Insights on the costs of school feeding compared with investments in primary education. Food Nutr Bull 34(3):310–317

18. Griebler R, Molcho M, Samdal O, Inchley J, Dur W, Currie C (2009) Health Behaviour in School-Aged Children: A World Health Organization Cross-national Study. Research protocol for the 2009–2010 survey. Vienna: LBPHIR and Edinburgh: CAHRU. http://www.hbsc.org

19. Hetland J, Torsheim T, Aarø LE (2002) Subjective health complaints in adolescence: dimensional structure and variation across gender and age. Scand J Public Health 30(3): 223–230

20. James WPT, Nelson M, Ralph A, Leather S (1997) The contribution of nutrition to inequalities in health. BMJ 314:1545–1549

21. Kyriakides L, Kaloyirou C, Lindsay G (2006) An analysis of the Revised Olweus Bully/Victim Questionnaire using the Rasch measurement model. Br J Educ Psychol 76:781–801

22. Longhurst R, Tomkins A (1995) The role of care in nutrition—a neglected essential ingredient. Cent Int Child Health Inst Child Health SCN News 12:60p

23. Melbye EL, Ogaard T, Overby NC, Hansen H (2013) Parental food-related behaviors and family meal frequencies: associations in Norwegian dyads of parents and preadolescent children. BMC Public Health 13:820

24. Melchior M, Chastang JF, Falissard B et al (2012) Food insecurity and children's mental health: a prospective birth cohort study. PLoS One 7(12):e52615

25. Molcho M, Gabhainn SN, Kelly C, Friel S, Kelleher C (2007) Food poverty and health among schoolchildren in Ireland: findings from the Health Behaviour in School-aged Children (HBSC) study. Public Health Nutr 10(4):64–370

26. Mullen E, Currie C, Boyce W, Morgan A, Kalnins I, Holstein B (2002) Social inequality. In: Currie C, Samdal O, Boyce W, Smith R (eds) Health Behaviour in School-aged Children: A World Health Organization Cross-national Study: Research Protocol for the 2001/02 survey. University of Edinburgh, Edinburgh

27. Nackers LM, Appelhans DM (2013) Food insecurity is linked to a food environment promoting obesity in households with children. Nutr Educ Behav 45(6):780–784

28. Nichol ME, Pickett W, Janssen I (2009) Associations between school recreational environments and physical activity. J School Health 79:247–254

29. Niclasen B, Molcho M, Arnfjord S, Schnohr C (2013a) Conceptualizing and contextualizing food insecurity among Greenlandic children. Int J Circumpolar Health 72:19928

30. Niclasen B, Petzold M, Schnohr CW (2013b) Adverse health effects of experiencing food insecurity among Greenlandic school children. Int J Circumpolar Health 72:20849

31. Pickett W, Molcho M, Elgar F et al (2013) Trends and socio-economic correlates of adolescent physical fighting in 30 countries. Pediatrics 131(1):e18–e26

32. Prochaska JJ, Sallis JF, Long B (2001) A physical activity screening measure for use with adolescents in primary care. Arch Pediatr Adolesc Med 155(5):554–559

33. Riches G (1997) Hunger, food security and welfare policies: issues and debates in first world societies. Proc Nutr Soc 56(1A):63–74

34. Robaina KA, Martin KS (2013) Food insecurity, poor diet quality, and obesity among food pantry participants in Hartford. CT. J Nutr Educ Behav 45(2):159–164

35. Statistics Canada (2014) Population by sex and age group. Ottawa: Statistics Canada, CANSIM, table 051-0001. http://www.statcan.gc.ca/tables-tableaux/sum-som/l01/cst01/demo10a-eng.htm, Accessed 22 Nov 2014

36. Stuff JE, Casey PH, Szeto KL et al (2004) Household food insecurity is associated with adult health status. J Nutr 134(9):2330–2335

37. Tarasuk V, Vogt J (2009) Household food insecurity in Ontario. Can J Public Health 100(3):184–188

38. United Nations (1959) Declaration of the rights of the child. Geneva: UN General Assembly: Resolution 1386 (XIV)

39. United Nations Children's Fund (1990) Strategy for improved nutrition of children and women in developing countries. UNICEF policy review, 1990–91 E/ICEF/1990/l.6. UNICEF, New York

40. Vozoris NT, Tarasuk VS (2003) Household food insufficiency is associated with poorer health. J Nutr 133(1):120–126

41. World Food Programme (2007) World Hunger Series 2007: hunger and health. London: earthscan. http://www.wfp.org/sites/default/files/World_Hunger_Series_2007_Hunger_and_Health_EN.pdf. Accessed 01 April 2014

CHAPTER 8

Food Insecurity and Children's Mental Health: A Prospective Birth Cohort Study

Maria Melchior, Jean-François Chastang,
Bruno Falissard, Cédric Galéra,
Richard E. Tremblay, Sylvana M. Côté,
and Michel Boivin

8.1 INTRODUCTION

In industrialized countries, approximately 5–15% of families experience food insecurity, that is insufficient access to "sufficient, safe, and nutritious food that meets individuals' dietary needs and preferences for an active and healthy life" [1]–[6]. Prior research has shown that food insecurity is associated with poor health and developmental outcomes in children [7]–[13]. In particular, children growing up in families that are food-insecure appear to have high levels of symptoms of anxiety/depression [12], [14]–[16], aggression, and hyperactivity/inattention [5], [12], [17]. This may be due to three mechanisms: 1) food insecurity may be associated with other exposures related to children's psychological well-being (e.g. low income); 2) food insecurity and children's mental health may have common causes (e.g. parental psychopathology); 3) food insecurity may independently predict children's psychological and behavioral well-being [18]; and 4) food insecurity may predict parental depression [19]. Thus, in order to examine associations between food insecurity and children's mental health, it is important to control for individual and familial characteristics which may confound this association.

Past research linking food insecurity to children's outcomes was mostly based on cross-sectional samples [5], [12], [14], [15] or short follow-up (up to two years) [16], [17] and the long-term consequences of exposure to food insecurity early on in life are not well known. In the present study, we test the relationship between food insecurity in early childhood (before age 4½) and children's symptoms of depression/anxiety, aggression, and hyperactivity/inattention up to age 8, accounting for child and familial characteristics which may be associated with food insecurity and children's mental health [16], [20]: child's sex, immigrant status, family structure, maternal age at child's birth, family income, maternal and paternal education, prenatal tobacco exposure, maternal and paternal depression, family functioning and negative parenting.

8.2   METHODS

Data for this study come from the Québec Longitudinal Study of Child Development (QLSCD) study, which follows a representative cohort of 2120 children born in the Canadian province of Québec in 1997–1998. To ensure geographic representation and minimize the effect of seasonality, participants were chosen through a random selection of children born throughout the year in each public health geographic area of the province. Twins and children with major diseases or handicaps at birth were excluded from the cohort. Selected children were first seen at 5 months of age and then once each year thereafter (follow-up assessments were conducted at 1½, 2½, 3½, 4½, 5, 6 and 8 years). Data on children and their parents were collected by trained interviewers through home interviews regularly conducted with the person most knowledgeable about the child (the mother in 98% of cases). Participating families gave written informed consent for the study at each assessment. The survey protocol was approved by the Quebec Institute of Statistics (Quebec City, Quebec, Canada) and the St-Justine Hospital Research Center (Montreal, Quebec, Canada) ethics committees. Informed consent for the study was obtained from parents or legal guardians.

The average response rate during the 8 years of data collection was 87.0% (range, 68%–100%) [20]. The present analysis is based on 1682 children with available data on food insecurity as well as at least 2 measures of mental health symptoms. Compared to the original cohort, nonparticipants were more likely to be from families that were characterized by low income, low education, immigrant background, young maternal age, single-parenthood and maternal depression, but participants and nonparticipants did not differ with regard to children's mental health symptoms.

8.2.1   Food Insecurity

Food insecurity was ascertained when the participating child was 1½ and 4½ years old. On those two occasions, mothers were asked: a) whether family members had eaten less than they should have because they had run out of food or money to buy food (1½ and 4½ years), b) whether family members had eaten the same foods several times because they did not have anything else and could not afford to buy other foods (4½ years only), c) whether the family could not afford to offer nutritious meals to the children (4½ years only), d) how often family members did not eat as much as they should have because they had run out of food or money to buy food (4½ years). These measures of food insecurity were previously shown to predict children's overweight and obesity [21], [22]. Children whose families experienced any of these situations were considered to be exposed to food insecurity: (3.4% of the study population at age 1½ year, 3.6% at age 4½ years, 5.9% at 1½ or 4½ years of age).

8.2.2   Children's Mental Health

Children's mental health was assessed at 4½, 5, 6 and 8 years based on parental reports. Symptoms of depression/anxiety were assessed using 5 items adapted from the Preschool Behavior Questionnaire [23] and the Child Behavioral Checklist [24]: 'nervous, high strung or tense', 'fearful or anxious', 'worried', 'not as happy as other children', 'has difficulty having fun' [25]. Symptoms of aggression were assessed using 5 items previously validated in this study: 'hits', 'kicks', 'bites', 'fights', 'bullies others' [26]. Symptoms of hyperactivity-impulsivity and inattention were assessed through a combination of items from the Child Behavior Checklist [24], the Ontario Child Health Study Scales [27] and the Preschool Behavior Questionnaire [28]. Hyperactivity-impulsivity was assessed using 5 items: 'can't sit still, is restless', 'fidgets', 'can't settle down to do anything for more than a few moments', 'is impulsive, acts without thinking', 'has difficulty waiting for turn in games' [29]. Inattention was assessed using 3 items:

"can't concentrate, can't pay attention for long", "is easily distracted, has trouble sticking to any activity", "is inattentive". All items pertaining to children's mental health symptoms were scored 0 ('never'), 1 ('sometimes') or 2 ('often') and then summed to range 0–10 [20].

Based on the four measures of children's psychological symptoms between ages 4½ and 8 years which were available to us, we used semiparametric mixture models [30] to calculate longitudinal symptom trajectories. This approach makes it possible to identify groups with distinct longitudinal symptom patterns empirically rather than using a set cut off. As such, this method provides a description of the 'natural' course of the evolution of mental health symptoms over time. Additionally, the reliance on multiple measures of symptoms as well as the grouping of children according to a trajectory pattern reduces the measurement in error related to a single assessment [31]. For each symptom group, the model implemented using the PROC TRAJ procedure in SAS defined the shape of the trajectory and the proportion of participants in each group. The validity of the 'best fitting" classification was confirmed using the Bayesian Information Criterion (BIC). Overall, we identified 3 groups of symptoms of depression/anxiety (low: 19.2%, moderate: 59.8%, high: 21.0%), 3 groups of symptoms of aggression (low: 23.8%, moderate/declining: 50.1%, high: 26.2%), and 4 groups of symptoms of hyperactivity/inattention, (low: 20.9%, low/intermediate: 38.3%, intermediate: 34.8%, high: 6.0%). Children's symptoms were moderately correlated to one another (correlation coefficients at age 8 years: depression/anxiety and aggression: 0.16, $p<0.0001$; depression/anxiety and hyperactivity/inattention: 0.31, $p<0.0001$; aggression and hyperactivity/inattention: 0.32, $p<0.0001$).

8.2.3   Covariates

Analyses were adjusted for the characteristics of children and their families, which can be associated with food insecurity and children's mental health symptoms [16]. Covariates were measured at age 5 months (prenatal tobacco exposure, maternal and paternal depressive symptoms and family functioning) or concomitantly to food insecurity. Demographics included the child's sex (male vs. female), immigrant status (immigrant vs. non-immigrant), family structure (parents separated vs. two-parent family) and maternal age at child's birth (<21 vs. >=21 years). Family income was calculated according to guidelines issued by Statistics Canada, taking into account the number of people in the household and the type of residence area (urban vs. rural based on population density);

family income was coded as insufficient vs. sufficient. Maternal and paternal education was defined as <High school vs. >=High school. Prenatal tobacco exposure was defined as maternal consumption of >=1 cigarette/day (yes vs. no). Maternal and paternal depressive symptoms were assessed by the abbreviated version (12 items) of the Center for Epidemiologic.

Studies Depression (CESD) Scale [32]. Parents reported the frequency of depressive symptoms in the previous week. Each item was coded on a 4-point scale. Total informant ratings were z-standardized. Family dysfunction was assessed with the McMaster Family Assessment, which includes 12 items measuring communication, showing and receiving affection, control of disruptive behaviour, and problem resolution in the family; each item was coded 0 ('never'), 1 ('sometimes'), or 2 ('often') and the overall score was z-standardized [33]. Negative parenting was assessed using the Parental Cognition and Conduct Toward the Infant Scale, which includes dimensions such as coercitive parenting (7 items) and overprotection (5 items), each rated on a scale ranging 0 to 10; overall scores were z-standardized [34].

8.2.4   Statistical Analysis

To study the association between food insecurity and children's mental health outcomes, we combined exposure to food insecurity when children were 1½ and 4½ years of age (ever food-insecure vs. never food-insecure) and tested associations with children's probability of being on a 'high' behavioural trajectory group at ages 4½ to 8 years. First, we tested sex-adjusted associations, in order to account for sex-related differences in the prevalence of mental health symptoms in children. Second, we adjusted for covariates. In additional analyses we tested whether the association between food insecurity and long-term behavioural problems 1) was robust to statistical adjustment on behavioural problems prior to age 4½; 2) differed depending on the child's sex. Analyses were carried out in a logistic regression framework in SAS (V9).

8.3   RESULTS

5.9% of study children experienced food insecurity between ages 1½ and 4½ years. As shown in Table 1, food insecurity was associated with characteristics of children and their families, including immigrant status, family structure, maternal age at child's birth, family income, maternal and paternal education,

TABLE 8.1 Characteristics of children and their families in relation to food insecurity: the Longitudinal Study of Child Development in Québec, 1997/98–2005.

	Food-insecure children n = 99	Non food-insecure children n = 1583	p-value
Children's characteristics			
Sex (%):	46.5	50.5	0.44
Female	53.5	49.5	
Male			
Immigrant status (%):	80.8	88.3	0.027
Non-immigrant	19.2	11.7	
Immigrant			
Symptoms of depression/anxiety:	10.1	19.8	0.0073
Low	58.6	59.8	
Intermediate	31.3	20.4	
High			
Symptoms of aggression:	18.2	24.1	0.35
Low	51.5	50.0	
Intermediate	30.3	25.9	
High			
Symptoms of hyperactivity/inattention:	17.2	21.1	0.0011
Low	37.4	38.3	
Low/intermediate	30.3	35.1	
Intermediate	15.2	5.4	
High			
Family characteristics			
Family structure (%):	49.5	77.2	<0.0001
Two-parent family	50.5	22.8	
Parents separated			
Maternal age at child's birth (%):	59.6	80.2	<0.0001
> = 21 years	40.4	19.8	
< 21 years			
Family income (%):	23.2	76.0	<0.0001
Sufficient	76.8	24.0	
Insufficient			

TABLE 8.1   *(Continued)*

	Food-insecure children n = 99	Non food-insecure children n = 1583	p-value
Maternal education (%):	33.7	15.4	<0.0001
< High school degree	66.3	84.6	
> = High school degree			
Paternal education (%):	46	18.4	<0.0001
< High school degree	54	81.6	
> = High school degree			
Prenatal tobacco exposure (%):	62.6	75.9	0.0030
No	37.4	24.1	
Yes			
Maternal depression score (μ, se)	2.24, 1.52	1.28, 1.07	<0.0001
Paternal depression score (μ, se)	1.33, 1.10	0.97, 0.94	0.0023
Family functionning score (μ, se)	0.27, 0.17	0.25, 0.15	0.18
Negative parenting score (μ, se)	3.28, 1.18	2.98, 1.02	0.0057

doi:10.1371/journal.pone.0052615.t001

prenatal tobacco exposure, maternal and paternal depression and negative parenting. In sex-adjusted regression analyses (Table 2), compared to unexposed children, children who experienced food insecurity were more likely to have persistently high levels of symptoms of depression/anxiety (OR: 1.79, 95% CI 1.15–2.79) and hyperactivity/inattention (OR: 3.06, 95% CI 1.68–5.55), but not aggression. In multivariate regression models adjusted for characteristics of children and their families (Table 3), the association between food insecurity and symptoms of depression/anxiety decreased and became statistically non-significant (fully adjusted OR: 1.44, 95% CI 0.78–2.66); however the association between food insecurity and symptoms of hyperactivity/inattention remained elevated and statistically significant (fully adjusted OR: 2.65, 95% CI 1.16–6.06). The decrease in ORs associated with food insecurity was greatest after controlling for maternal depression (41% for symptoms of depression/anxiety and 42% for symptoms of hyperactivity/inattention). In additional analyses further adjusted for hyperactivity/inattention at age 1½ years, the association between food insecurity and hyperactivity/inattention between ages 4½ and 8 years remained elevated but lost statistical significance (OR: 2.18, 95%

CI 0.60–8.00). Sex-stratified analyses showed no significant differences in the association between food insecurity and hyperactivity/inattention in boys and girls and the interaction test was not statistically significant (p=0.88).

TABLE 8.2 Food insecurity and children's characteristics in relation to trajectories of psychological difficulties ages 4–8 years: the Longitudinal Study of Child Development in Québec, 1997/98–2005 (sex-adjusted ORs, 95% CI).

	High depression/ anxiety prevalence: 21.0% OR (95% CI)	High aggression prevalence: 26.2% OR (95% CI)	High hyperactivity/ inattention prevalence: 6.0% OR (95% CI)
Food insecurity :	1	1	1
No	1.79 (1.15–2.79)	1.21 (0.77–1.90)	3.06 (1.68–5.55)
Yes			
Immigrant status:	1	1	1
Non-immigrant	0.90 (0.63–1.30)	0.91 (0.64–1.28)	0.89 (0.47–1.70)
Immigrant			
Family structure:	1	1	1
Two-parent family	1.11 (0.85–1.45)	1.52 (1.19–1.95)	2.54 (1.67–3.85)
Parents separated			
Maternal age at child's birth:	1	1	1
> = 21 years	0.93 (0.69–1.25)	1.55 (1.20–2.02)	2.33 (1.51–3.59)
< 21 years			
Family income:	1	1	1
Sufficient	1.28 (0.99–1.65)	1.40 (1.10–1.78)	2.11 (1.40–3.19)
Insufficient			
Maternal education:	1	1	1
> = High school degree	1.08 (0.79–1.47]	1.42 (1.07–1.90)	1.80 (1.12–2.90)
< High school degree			
Paternal education:	1	1	1
> = High school degree	1.08 (0.79–1.46)	1.80 (1.37–2.37)	2.87 (1.81–4.54)
< High school degree			
Prenatal tobacco exposure:	1	1	1
No	0.88 (0.67–1.16)	1.60 (1.25–2.04)	1.96 (1.28–3.00)
Yes			

TABLE 8.2 *(Continued)*

	High depression/ anxiety prevalence: 21.0% OR (95% CI)	High aggression prevalence: 26.2% OR (95% CI)	High hyperactivity/ inattention prevalence: 6.0% OR (95% CI)
Maternal depression score (per unit)	1.25 (1.14–1.38)	1.22 (1.11–1.34)	1.43 (1.24–1.64)
Paternal depression score (per unit)	1.11 (0.98–1.26)	1.12 (1.00–1.27)	1.26 (1.03–1.54)
Family functionning score (per unit)	1.70 (0.81–3.60)	2.68 (1.34–5.37)	2.86 (0.85–9.66)
Negative parenting score (per unit)	1.46 (1.30–1.63)	1.75 (1.56–1.96)	1.88 (1.57–2.26)

doi:10.1371/journal.pone.0052615.t002.

TABLE 8.3 Food insecurity and children's trajectories of psychological difficulties ages 4–8 years: the Longitudinal Study of Child Development in Québec, 1997/98–2005 (multivariate ORs, 95% CI; beta, se)[1]

	High depression/ anxiety OR (95% CI)	High aggression OR (95% CI)	High hyperactivity/ inattention OR (95% CI)
Food insecurity :	1	1	1
No	1.44 (0.78–2.66)	0.67 (0.35–1.29)	2.65 (1.16–6.06)
Yes			
Sex:	1	1	1
Female	0.80 (0.62–1.05)	2.07 (1.59–2.69)	2.46 (1.43–4.23)
Male			
Immigrant status:	1	1	1
Non-immigrant	0.65 (0.42–1.02)	0.79 (0.52–1.20)	0.69 (0.30–1.60)
Immigrant			
Family structure:	1	1	1
Two parent family	1.04 (0.72–1.50)	1.25 (0.89–1.77)	1.36 (0.74–2.49)
Parents separated			
Maternal age at child's birth:	1	1	1
> = 21 years	0.94 (0.64–1.40)	1.25 (0.87–1.81)	1.55 (0.83–2.90)
< 21 years			
Family income:	1	1	1
Sufficient	1.05 (0.73–1.52)	1.05 (0.74–1.50)	0.90 (0.47–1.72)
Insufficient			

TABLE 8.3 *(Continued)*

	High depression/ anxiety OR (95% CI)	High aggression OR (95% CI)	High hyperactivity/ inattention OR (95% CI)
Maternal education:	1	1	1
> = High school degree	1.25 (0.82–1.91)	0.98 (0.65–1.48)	0.77 (0.36–1.64)
< High school degree			
Paternal education:	1	1	1
> = High school degree	0.88 (0.61–1.28)	1.51 (1.07–2.11)	1.80 (1.00–3.24)
< High school degree			
Prenatal tobacco exposure:	1	1	1
No	0.68 (0.48–0.96)	1.18 (0.86–1.62)	1.11 (0.61–2.00)
Yes			
Maternal depression score (per unit)	1.23 (1.08–1.39)	1.13 (1.00–1.28)	1.22 (0.99–1.51)
Paternal depression score (per unit)	1.03 (0.89–1.18)	1.03 (0.90–1.19)	1.12 (0.88–1.43)
Family functionning score (per unit)	1.93 (0.77–4.81)	2.68 (1.13–6.37)	1.15 (0.23–5.87)
Negative parenting score (per unit)	1.42 (1.24–1.62)	1.70 (1.49–1.93)	1.75 (1.39–2.20)

8.4 DISCUSSION

In a birth cohort study of families with young children followed for up to 8 years, we found that food insecurity predicted children's two-fold increase in the likelihood of persistent hyperactivity/inattention, even after accounting for family socioeconomic circumstances and parental mental health, although this association lost statistical significance when further adjusted for children's behavioural symptoms at age 1½ years. To our knowledge, this is the first study to examine the relationship between food insecurity and children's mental health over such an extended follow-up, independently of individual and family characteristics known to predict children's outcomes. Our finding contributes to growing scientific evidence of the impact of food insecurity on children's well-being, and suggests that exposure very early in life can have lasting effects on development.

8.4.1   Limitations and Strengths

Prior to discussing the study findings, we need to acknowledge methodological limitations: 1) due to selective attrition which often occurs in longitudinal cohort studies, the study sample included fewer children from socioeconomically disadvantaged families than the original cohort; thus, the prevalence of food insecurity among Canadian families with small children may be higher than we report; 2) children were not assessed for clinically significant emotional and behavioural problems, barring conclusions regarding the impact of food insecurity on psychological problems that require medical attention; nevertheless, children who experience mental health difficulties early on are at risk of psychiatric disorders later in life implying that symptoms such as the ones we measured require attention from parents, teachers and physicians [35]; 3) children's mental health symptoms were assessed by their mothers, raising the possibility of reporting bias, particularly if the mother was depressed; evidence that maternal reports of children's behaviour coincide with reports of other individuals in children's environment (father, other family, friends) [25], [36], [37] implies that symptoms picked up by mothers are valid; nevertheless future investigations should account for teacher ratings, particularly to measure hyperactivity/inattention, as a way to alleviate problems related to potential shared method variance; 4) food insecurity was measured using four items, which may have led us to underestimate its occurrence as not all aspects of food shortage and inadequacy were assessed; additionally, we did not have sufficient statistical power to study children's mental health in relation to changes in food insecurity over time.

Our study also has key strengths: 1) analyses were based on a community sample and we were able to estimate the burden of behavioural problems associated with food insecurity among children in the general population, while most prior studies focused on high-risk families; 2) longitudinal follow-up of children's mental health allowed us to distinguish different types of symptoms and their developmental patterns over up to 7 years of follow-up; 3) statistical adjustment for multiple individual and family factors potentially associated with children's outcomes.

8.4.2   Food Insecurity and Children's Behaviour

Our finding of an association between exposure to food insecurity and children's mental health symptoms is consistent with prior research conducted cross-sectionally or over a limited follow-up [5], [12], [38]. In contrast to studies conducted in high-risk [12], [14] or older samples [15], [16], the association between food insecurity and children's symptoms of emotional problems in our study disappeared after we adjusted for individual and family factors.

Adding to prior research which did not always distinguish specific aspects of children's behaviour, we found that food insecurity is distinctively associated with children's symptoms of hyperactivity/inattention. This association lost statistical significance after adjusting for children's behavioural difficulties at age 1½ years, but did not much change, which may be due to the small number of cases of hyperactivity/inattention in our study and calls for additional research in larger samples.

The association between food insecurity and children's behaviour may reflect several mechanisms. First, food insecure families are disproportionately exposed to multiple risks which can impair children's development and mental health, including poverty, marital discord, single parenthood, violence, parental substance abuse and psychopathogy [39], [40]. Our analyses are controlled for income, family structure and functioning, as well as parental psychopathology and attitude towards children, but we cannot entirely rule out the possibility of residual confounding, whereby the association between food insecurity and children's behaviour is not causal but rather reflects the co-occurrence of other risk factors. Second, through psychological pathways, food insecurity early in life may lead to weak attachment between parents and children, which can have negative consequences on children's mental health later on [41]. Third, food insecurity may be associated with maternal depression, which, in turn, impacts on child mental health [19]. Fourth, food insecurity may directly predict the occurrence of behavioural difficulties through inadequate nutrition [18]. In particular, compared to non food-insecure children, food-insecure children's diets are high in fat, refined sugars and sodium and low in fruits, vegetables and fiber [42], leading to high carbohydrate intake [43] and decreased levels of vitamin, omega-3, fatty acids and iron [44], [45]. High consumption of refined sugars as well as iron-deficiency anaemia may have behavioural consequences such as hyperkinesia, inattention and poor memory, and may contribute to the link between food insecurity and hyperactivity/inattention. Although there is controversy regarding the importance of dietary factors in relation to ADHD risk, recent evidence from intervention trials suggests that the introduction of a healthy diet yields improvements in symptoms in some children [46], [47]. Given the burden of ADHD in children and adults [48], and the impact of hyperactivity/inattention on children's concurrent and future health, academic, and social outcomes [49]–[51], ensuring children's mental health should be a public health priority.

8.5 CONCLUSIONS

Children growing up in food-insecure families are two-times more likely to have high levels of persistent symptoms of hyperactivity/inattention than children who are not food insecure. Reducing the burden of food insecurity in families could help decrease the burden of mental health problems in school-aged children and reduce social inequalities in development.

REFERENCES

1. Food and Agriculture Organization of the United Nations (2003) Trade reforms and food security.
2. Che J, Chen J (2001) Food insecurity in Canadian households. Health Rep 12: 11–22.
3. Evenson KR, Laraia BA, Welch VL, Perry AL (2002) Statewide prevalences of concern about enough food, 1996–1999. Public Health Rep 117: 358–365. doi: 10.1016/s0033-3549(04)50172-3
4. Molcho M, Gabhainn SN, Kelly C, Friel S, Kelleher C (2007) Food poverty and health among schoolchildren in Ireland: findings from the Health Behaviour in School-aged Children (HBSC) study. Public Health Nutr 10: 364–370. doi: 10.1017/s1368980007226072
5. Melchior M, Caspi A, Howard L, Ambler AP, Bolton H, et al. (2009) The mental health context of food insecurity in families with young children. Pediatrics 24: e564–e572. doi: 10.1542/peds.2009-0583
6. Martin-Fernandez J, Caillavet F, Chauvin P (2011) L'insécurité alimentaire dans l'agglomération parisienne: prévalence et inégalités socio-territoriales. Bull Epidémiol Hebd 515–521.
7. Jyoti DF, Frongillo EA, Jones SJ (2005) Food insecurity affects school children's academic performance, weight gain, and social skills. J Nutr 135: 2831–2839.
8. Rose D, Bodor JN (2006) Household food insecurity and overweight status in young school children: results from the Early Childhood Longitudinal Study. Pediatrics 117: 464–473. doi: 10.1542/peds.2005-0582
9. Whitaker RC, Phillips SM, Orzol SM (2006) Food insecurity and the risks of depression and anxiety in mothers and behavior problems in their preschool-aged children. Pediatrics 118: e859–e868. doi: 10.1542/peds.2006-0239
10. Casey P, Goolsby S, Berkowitz C, Frank D, Cook J, et al. (2004) Maternal depression, changing public assistance, food security, and child health status. Pediatrics 113: 298–304. doi: 10.1542/peds.113.2.298
11. Broughton MA, Janssen PS, Hertzman C, Innis SM, Frankish CJ (2006) Predictors and outcomes of household food insecurity among inner city families with preschool children in Vancouver. Can J Public Health 97: 214–216.
12. Kleinman RE, Murphy JM, Little M, Pagano M, Wehler CA, et al. (1998) Hunger in children in the United States: potential behavioral and emotional correlates. Pediatrics 101: E3. doi: 10.1542/peds.101.1.e3

13. Alaimo K, Olson CM, Frongillo EA (2001) Food insufficiency and American school-aged children's cognitive, academic, and psychosocial development. Pediatrics 108: 44–53.

14. Weinreb L, Wehler C, Perloff J, Scott R, Hosmer D, et al. (2002) Hunger: its impact on children's health and mental health. Pediatrics 110: e41. doi: 10.1542/peds.110.4.e41

15. Alaimo K, Olson CM, Frongillo EA (2002) Family food insufficiency, but not low family income, is positively associated with dysthymia and suicide symptoms in adolescents. J Nutr 132: 719–725.

16. Belsky DW, Moffitt TE, Arseneault L, Melchior M, Caspi A (2010) Context and sequelae of food insecurity in children's development. Am J Epidemiol 172: 809–818. kwq201 [pii];10.1093/aje/kwq201 [doi].

17. Murphy JM, Wehler CA, Pagano ME, Little M, Kleinman RE, et al. (1998) Relationship between hunger and psychosocial functioning in low-income American children. J Am Acad Child Adolesc Psychiatry 37: 163–170. doi: 10.1097/00004583-199802000-00008

18. Ashiabi G, O'Neal K (2008) A framework for understanding the association between food insecurity and children's developmental outcomes. Child Development Perspectives 2: 71–77. doi: 10.1111/j.1750-8606.2008.00049.x

19. Bronte-Tinkew J, Zaslow M, Capps R, Horowitz A, McNamara M (2007) Food insecurity works through depression, parenting, and infant feeding to influence overweight and health in toddlers. J Nutr 137: 2160–2165.

20. Galéra C, Côté SM, Bouvard MP, Pingault JB, Melchior M, et al. (2011) Early risk factors for hyperactivity-impulsivity and inattention trajectories from age 17 months to 8 years. Arch Gen Psychiatry 68: 1267–1275. doi: 10.1001/archgenpsychiatry.2011.138

21. Dubois L, Farmer A, Girard M, Porcherie M (2006) Family food insufficiency is related to overweight among preschoolers. Soc Sci Med 63: 1503–1516. doi: 10.1016/j.socscimed. 2006.04.002

22. Dubois L, Francis D, Burnier D, Tatone-Tokuda F, Girard M, et al. (2011) Household food insecurity and childhood overweight in Jamaica and Quebec: a gender-based analysis. BMC Public Health 11: 199. doi: 10.1186/1471-2458-11-199

23. Behar L, Stringfield S (1974) A behavior rating scale for the preschool child. Develop Psychol 10: 601–610. doi: 10.1037/h0037058

24. Achenbach Thomas (1991) Manual for the child behavior checklist/4–18. Burlington, VT: University of Vermont Department of Psychology.

25. Côté SM, Boivin M, Liu X, Nagin DS, Zoccolillo M, et al. (2009) Depression and anxiety symptoms: onset, developmental course and risk factors during early childhood. J Child Psychol Psychiatry 50: 1201–1208. doi: 10.1111/j.1469-7610.2009.02099.x

26. Côté SM, Boivin M, Nagin DS, Japel C, Xu Q, et al. (2007) The role of maternal education and nonmaternal care services in the prevention of children's physical aggression problems. Arch Gen Psychiatry 64: 1305–1312. doi: 10.1001/archpsyc.64.11.1305

27. Boyle MH, Offord DR, Racine Y, Sanford M, Szatmari P, et al. (1993) Evaluation of the original Ontario Child Health Study scales. Can J Psychiatry 38: 397–405. doi: 10.1111/ j.1469-7610.1993.tb00979.x

28. Tremblay RE, Desmarais-Gervais L, Gagnon C, Charlebois P (1987) The Preschool Behavior Questionnaire: Stability of its factor structure between cultures, sexes, ages and socioeconomic classes. Int J Behav Develop 10: 467–484. doi: 10.1177/016502548701000406

29. Huijbregts SC, Seguin JR, Zoccolillo M, Boivin M, Tremblay RE (2008) Maternal prenatal smoking, parental antisocial behavior, and early childhood physical aggression. Develop Psychopathol 20: 437–453. doi: 10.1017/s0954579408000217

30. Jones BL, Nagin DS, Roeder K (2001) A SAS procedure based on mixture models for estimating developmental trajectories. Sociol Methods Res 29: 374–393. doi: 10.1177/0049124101029003005

31. Nagin DS, Odgers CL (2010) Group-Based Trajectory Modeling (Nearly) Two Decades Later. J Quant Criminol 26: 445–453. doi: 10.1007/s10940-010-9113-7

32. Radloff L (1977) The CES-D scale: a self report depression scale for research in the general population. Appl Psychological Measurement 1: 385–401. doi: 10.1177/014662167700100306

33. Statistics Canada (1995) Overview of Survey Instruments for 1994–1995 Data Collection, Cycle 1.

34. Boivin M, Pérusse D, Dionne G, Saysset V, Zoccolillo M, et al. (2005) The genetic-environmental etiology of parents' perceptions and self-assessed behaviours toward their 5-month-old infants in a large twin and singleton sample. J Child Psychol Psychiatry 46: 612–630. doi: 10.1111/j.1469-7610.2004.00375.x

35. Rutter M, Kim-Cohen J, Maughan B (2006) Continuities and discontinuities in psychopathology between childhood and adult life. J Child Psychol Psychiatry 47: 276–295. doi: 10.1111/j.1469-7610.2006.01614.x

36. Cicchetti D, Toth SL (1998) The development of depression in children and adolescents. Am Psychol 53: 221–241. doi: 10.1037/0003-066x.53.2.221

37. Baumann B, William E, Lang A, Jacob R, Blumenthal J (2004) The impact of maternal depressive symptomatology on ratings of children with ADHD and child confederates. J Emotion Behav Disord 12: 90–98. doi: 10.1177/10634266040120020301

38. Murphy JM, Pagano ME, Nachmani J, Sperling P, Kane S, et al. (1998) The relationship of school breakfast to psychosocial and academic functioning: cross-sectional and longitudinal observations in an inner-city school sample. Arch Pediatr Adolesc Med 152: 899–907. doi: 10.1001/archpedi.152.9.899

39. Health consequences of poverty for children. End child poverty. Available: http://www.endchildpoverty.org.uk/files/Health_consequences_of_Poverty_for_children pdf. Accessed 2012 April 30.

40. Ashiabi GS, O'Neal KK (2007) Children's health status: examining the associations among income poverty, material hardship, and parental factors. PLoS ONE 2: e940. doi: 10.1371/journal.pone.0000940

41. Zaslow M, Bronte-Tinkew J, Capps R, Horowitz A, Moore KA, et al. (2009) Food security during infancy. implications for attachment and mental proficiency in toddlerhood. Mat Child Health J 13: 66–80. doi: 10.1007/s10995-008-0329-1

42. Pilgrim A, Barker M, Jackson A, Ntani G, Crozier S, et al. (2011) Does living in a food insecure household impact on the diets and body composition of young children? Findings from the Southampton Women's Survey. J Epidemiol Community Health. jech.2010.125476 [pii];10.1136/jech.2010.125476 [doi].

43. Casey PH, Szeto K, Lensing S, Bogle M, Weber J (2001) Children in food-insufficient, low-income families: prevalence, health, and nutrition status. Arch Pediatr Adolesc Med 155: 508–514. pnu00206 [pii].

44. Rose D (1999) Economic determinants and dietary consequences of food insecurity in the United States. J Nutr 129: 517S–520S.

45. Millichap JG, Yee MM (2012) The diet factor in attention-deficit/hyperactivity disorder. Pediatrics 129: 330–337. doi: 10.1542/peds.2011-2199

46. McCann D, Barrett A, Cooper A, Crumpler D, Dalen L, et al. (2007) Food additives and hyperactive behaviour in 3-year-old and 8/9-year-old children in the community: a randomised, double-blinded, placebo-controlled trial. Lancet 370: 1560–1567. S01-6736(07)613-3 [pii];10.1016/S01-6736(07)613-3 [doi].

47. Pelsser LM, Frankena K, Toorman J, Savelkoul HF, Dubois AE, et al. (2011) Effects of a restricted elimination diet on the behaviour of children with attention-deficit hyperactivity disorder (INCA study): a randomised controlled trial. Lancet 377: 494–503. S0140-6736(10)62227-1 [pii];10.1016/S0140-6736(10)62227-1 [doi].

48. Polanczyk G, Rohde LA (2007) Epidemiology of attention-deficit/hyperactivity disorder across the lifespan. Curr Opin Psychiatry 20: 386–392. doi: 10.1097/yco.0b013e3281568d7a

49. Galéra C, Bouvard MP, Messiah A, Fombonne E (2008) Hyperactivity-inattention symptoms in childhood and substance use in adolescence: The Youth Gazel cohort. Drug Alcohol Depend 94: 30–37. doi: 10.1016/j.drugalcdep.2007.09.022

50. Galéra C, Melchior M, Chastang JF, Bouvard MP, Fombonne E (2009) Childhood and adolescent hyperactivity-inattention symptoms and academic achievement 8 years later: the GAZEL Youth study. Psycholo Med 9: 1895–1906. doi: 10.1017/s0033291709005510

51. Galéra C, Bouvard M-P, Lagarde E, Touchette E, Fombonne E, et al. (2012) Attention problems in childhood and socioeconomic disadvantage 18 years later: the TEMPO cohort. Br J Psychiatry [In press].

PART IV
Food Security and Child Obesity

CHAPTER 9

Household Food Insecurity and Childhood Overweight in Jamaica and Québec: A Gender-Based Analysis

Lise Dubois, Damion Francis, Daniel Burnier, Fabiola Tatone-Tokuda, Manon Girard, Georgiana Gordon-Strachan, Kristin Fox, and Rainford Wilks

9.1 BACKGROUND

In most countries where data are available, the prevalence of childhood overweight has increased [1] to the point of becoming a major public health problem. Although there is some indication that this epidemic may be leveling-off in certain countries over recent years, this evidence is less apparent in lower-SES groups and does not seem to be the case for Canada and some European and Asian countries [2]. Childhood overweight is also associated with numerous short and long-term physiological and psychosocial negative health consequences in both individuals and populations [3–6]. Some studies purport that the epidemic of overweight is due to an increased consumption of low-nutrient, energy-dense products that are high in sugar and fats [7–11]. Others suggest that weight increases are mainly attributable to physical inactivity [10, 11].

The childhood overweight epidemic is not restricted to developed countries: a number of lower- and middle-income countries have been struggling with the double burden of underweight and overweight for some time [12, 13]. In urban areas of countries undergoing rapid social and economic change (e.g., China, Mexico, Egypt, and Brazil), the prevalence of overweight among children has reached levels comparable to those in developed countries [14]. In western developed countries, childhood adiposity has, for the most part, been shown to inversely associate with socioeconomic status (SES), according to a systematic review of studies from 1990-2005 [15]; whereas, in developing countries, a greater prevalence of childhood overweight has been observed in higher socioeconomic groups [1]. Some gender differences in this association have been noted, however. A seminal review of 144 published studies on the association between SES and overweight/obesity found a strong inverse relationship particularly among women in developed societies; this relationship was inconsistent for men and children. In developing countries, however, a direct association was observed between SES and obesity among men, women, and children [16, 17], although a high prevalence of obesity has been reported even among very poor women in developing countries [18].

Another public health problem that concerns both developing and, to a lesser extent, developed countries is food insecurity. Food insecurity arises when individuals do not have sufficient access to safe and nutritious foods at all times, to sustain active and healthy lives [19]. Some studies have reported a paradoxical positive association between food insecurity and childhood obesity [20–22]. However, there have been some inconsistent findings in this research area, with some studies reporting a negative association [23–25] or completely non-existent association between food insecurity and childhood obesity [26, 27].

Thus, this study aims, firstly, to examine whether household food insecurity is significantly related to child overweight/obesity in the Canadian province of Québec (total population of less than 8 million) and in the country of Jamaica (total population less than 3 million) and, secondly, to explore gender differences in the association between food insecurity and overweight/obesity in both polities. This study is part of an ongoing collaboration between the University of the West Indies' Epidemiology Research Unit (based in Kingston, Jamaica) and the Institute of Population Health (University of Ottawa, Canada). The prevalence of childhood overweight/obesity is high in both Canada and Jamaica: 26% of 6-to-11-year-old Canadian children were overweight or obese in 2004 according to the age- and sex-specific criteria developed by the International Obesity Task Force [28]; while, in Jamaica, the prevalence of overweight in 11-to-12-year-old children living in the Kingston Metropolitan area was reported to be 19% (BMI ≥ 85th percentile) in 1998 [29]. Furthermore, data from the Canadian Community Health Survey revealed that approximately 7% of Québec households were food-insecure in 2007-2008 [30]. Data on the prevalence of food insecurity among Jamaican households, however, has yet to be published. For the present study, it was hypothesized that a positive association would be observed between household food insecurity and childhood overweight/obesity in Québec, while a negative association would be observed in Jamaica, independent from other factors potentially associated with child overweight/ obesity.

9.2 METHODS

9.2.1 Background on Study Samples

9.2.1.1 Québec

Analyses were conducted using data from the Québec Longitudinal Study of Child Development (QLSCD), a study conducted by Santé Québec, a division of the Institut de la Statistique du Québec (ISQ) [31]. Approval from the Ministry of Health Ethics Committee and consent from participants were obtained. The QLSCD, established to examine the role of familial and social factors in children's health, cognitive, and behavioural development, followed a representative sample (n = 2103) of children born in 1998, in the province of Québec (approximately 70,000 newborns per year), Canada. To ensure geographic representation and minimize the effect of seasonality, the study randomly selected children born throughout the year in each public health geographic area of the province. A public health geographic area or "health region" refers to a geographic unit defined by the provincial ministry of health. Health regions facilitate public health administration for Canadians. Children and their parents were first seen at 5 months (gestational age adjusted for preterm birth) and at one-year intervals thereafter. Standardized, questionnaire-based face-to-face interviews and self-administered questionnaires, completed by the children's mothers and fathers, were used at each cycle of data-collection. Data pertaining to the child was obtained from the person deemed most knowledgeable about the child, which generally was the mother. Information was also obtained from the child's medical records. Of the 2103 infants included in the first cycle of the study, 1190 children remained in the study 10 years later, in 2008.

9.2.1.2   Jamaica

Jamaican data were drawn from the Jamaica Youth Risk and Resiliency Behaviour Survey 2005, conducted by the University of the West Indies [32]. The main purpose of this cross-sectional survey was to monitor the health status, nutritional habits, and lifestyles of children and young teenagers aged 10-15 years, in a nationally representative sample of Jamaican children currently enrolled in school, and to examine how these variables relate to demographic and socio-economic factors. The data were obtained from the children using trained interviewers who administered questionnaires which were standardized and validated for use in this population. Most children attended primary or secondary schools regularly. The average daily rate of attendance for primary school children was 78.5% [33, 34]. Enrolment records, obtained from the Ministry of Education, Youth and Culture, and school attendance registers from selected schools provided the sample frames used in this study.

A multi-stage random sampling method was employed. The first stage involved the random selection of schools within each region where probability was proportional to size. The second stage entailed randomly selecting children from grades within the required age groups. The number of schools selected and the number of students selected per school were proportional to the total number of children in the required age group per parish and school. In 2003, there were 279,986 children in the 10-to-14-year age group and 250,352 in the 15-to-19-year age group. These combined represented approximately 20% of the Jamaican population [35]. Using information on the rate of tobacco use among youths aged 10 to 14 (19%) [36], a confidence level of 95% and an error of + 2% yielded a required sample size of 2,500 children (EPI-Info software obtained from the Centers for Disease Control and Prevention [CDC] website). Based on an expected refusal rate of 10%, the sample size was adjusted to 2,800. For this analysis, 1674 children between ages 10 and 11 years were selected for study.

9.2.2   Measures

9.2.2.1   Overweight and Obesity

In Québec, children's heights and weights were measured at home by a trained interviewer following a standardized protocol using a measuring tape, ruler, and scale [37] when children were 10 years old. In Jamaica, body weight, without shoes and with light clothing, was recorded to the nearest 0.1 kg using a calibrated electronic platform scale. Standing height was recorded to the nearest 0.1 cm using a Leicester portable measuring rod. Measurements were obtained at school by trained interviewers following a standardized study protocol. Body mass index (BMI) was calculated as body weight/height2 (kg/m^2). Overweight and obesity were similarly defined in Québec and Jamaica according to Cole's criteria, which provide age- and sex-specific cut-off points for overweight and obesity in children between 2 and 18 years of age [38].

9.2.2.2 Food Insecurity

Food insecurity was assessed in comparable ways in Québec and Jamaica, and fit within the definitional ambits adopted by both the Food and Agriculture Organization (FAO) and the United States Department of Agriculture (USDA) [19, 39, 40]. In the Québec sample, data on food insecurity were collected via self-administered questionnaires addressed to mothers when children were 10 years of age. Using a 3-point Likert-type scale (rated "Often true", "Sometimes true", "Never true"), mothers were asked to rate how often their families had experienced each of the three following situations: 1) *We eat the same thing several days in a row because we only have a few different kinds of food on hand, and don't have enough money to buy more*; 2) *We eat less than we should because we don't have enough money for food*; and 3) *We can't provide balanced meals for our children because we can't afford it financially*. Children were classified as living in a food-insecure household if mothers answered "often true" or "sometimes true" to any of the three food insecurity statements, and as living in a food-secure household if mothers answered "never true" to each statement.

In the Jamaican sample, children were interviewed to ascertain the presence or absence of food insecurity as well as the extent to which they were food-insecure using two structured questions. The first dichotomous question was: 1) *During a usual week, do you go hungry because there is not enough food in your home?* (rated "Yes" or "No") Children were categorized as being food-insecure if they answered yes to question 1. They were then asked how often they experienced hunger using a 4-point Likert-type rating scale to categorize the extent of food insecurity: 2) *During a usual week, how often do you go hungry because there was not enough food in your home?* (rated "Always", "Most of the time", "Sometimes", "Rarely"). This method of combining responses has been employed in other studies on food-insecurity [41, 42]. In both questionnaires, the food-insecurity statements gather information at the household level, which has been demonstrated to have both face validity [43, 44] and external validity [45, 46].

9.2.2.3   Diet and Physical Activity

In Québec, food consumption (daily consumption of pastries, fruits, and vegetables) was measured by way of a self-administered Food Frequency Questionnaire (FFQ) completed by the children's mothers when the children were 10 years old. The children's mothers were asked: *In the past week, at home and at school (or school's daycare service), on average, how many times during the week or how many times per day has your child eaten the following foods.* The mothers chose one of the following responses: "none", "one to two times per week", "three to four times per week", "five to six times per week", "one time per day", "twice per day", "three times per day", or "four or more times per day". Daily consumption of pastries included pastries, candies, cookies, chips, and chewing gum containing sugar. Daily consumption of fruits excluded the consumption of fruit drinks or juice. Vegetable consumption included potatoes. Parents reported children's level of physical activity by stating whether their child had a "higher" or "much higher" level of physical activity in comparison to other children, or "same", "lower" or "much lower" level than other children. Children's level of physical activity was reported by the parents at age 6. All other variables included in the present study were completed when the children were 10 years old.

In Jamaica, children provided information about their dietary consumption patterns throughout a usual week (i.e., a week without social events that might affect usual intake). A standard questionnaire was validated for use in similar populations of adolescents [47]. Two questions were asked specifically about fruit consumption: (1) *During a usual week, do you eat fruit such as mango, orange, and pawpaw?* Response categories for this first question were: "yes", "no" and "don't know". If the child's response was "yes", then the interviewer proceeded to the following question: (2) *During a usual week, how many times per week do you usually eat fruit, such as mango, orange, and pawpaw?* Response categories were "<1, 1, 2, 3, 4, 5 or more, and don't know". A similarly structured set of questions was asked about usual weekly and daily consumption of vegetables (which did not include potatoes) and pastries (cake, bulla cake, buns, etc.). Physical activity was assessed using the short form of the International Physical Activity Questionnaire (IPAQ) [48] for leisure time physical activity, and children's level of physical activity was classified as "none or low" or "moderate or high".

9.2.2.4   Family Type and Socioeconomic Status (Ses)

In Québec, the SES index was calculated by the Institut de la Statistique du Québec [49] based on methods developed by Willms and Shields (1996) that aggregate annual gross income, education level, and occupational prestige for both parents [50]. SES was less rigorously defined in the Jamaican sample due to the unavailability of data: it was based on household crowding terciles and a geographical index (urban, rural, remote rural) developed by the Statistical Institute of Jamaica (STATIN). These two variables were combined to derive a proxy for SES. Family type categories were two-parent family, blended family, and single-parent family in both the Québec and Jamaican samples.

9.2.3   Statistical Analyses

Statistical analyses were conducted using SAS (version 9.2; SAS Institute; Cary, NC) and Stata (Version 10.1 Stata Corp.). In Québec, data were weighted by a factor based on the inverse of the selection probability, the probability of non-response, and the post-stratification and attrition rates to ensure that the data were longitudinally representative of infants born in 1998, in the province of Québec [51]. The weights used were provided by the Institut de la Statistique du Québec and included corrections for response bias. Thus, the rates obtained through this study are comparable to those from other surveys on the same population that use weighted responses, independent of the distribution of the sample [37]. The Jamaican data were weighted by age, sex, school type, and parish to provide normalized weights using data from STATIN.

Univariate associations were verified by performing a chi-square test on contingency tables. The significance level was set at 5%, and significant independent variables and other putative explanatory variables were included in multivariate analyses. Based on the literature, children's sex, level of physical activity, family type, family SES (by tertile: low, medium, high), and children's daily consumption of fruit, vegetables, and pastries were considered potential confounders. Our final models included food insecurity, SES, and family type.

In the Québec model, adjustments were made for pastry and vegetable consumption (significantly associated in the univariate analysis) and physical activity (due to its integral role in the equation of energy balance). The Jamaican model was adjusted for physical activity (significantly associated in the univariate analysis). Kendall Tau's test for correlation was also employed to ensure that SES and household food insecurity were not highly correlated and could be included in the same model as independent variables. Odds ratio (OR) estimates, with 95% confidence intervals, were computed using logistic regressions. The impact of missing data was assessed by conducting with-and-without analyses, which revealed no effect on the outcomes and results seen.

9.3   RESULTS

Characteristics of the Québec and Jamaican children are presented in Table 1. Approximately one-quarter (26%) of children from Québec and one-tenth (11%) of children from Jamaica were overweight or obese. Food insecurity was reported for 9% of the children in Québec and 26% in Jamaica. A greater proportion of children lived in single-parent families in Jamaica (36%) in comparison to Québec (17%). Fruit and vegetable consumption was higher in Québec than in Jamaica, whereas the difference in physical activity was less marked.

TABLE 9.1   A comparison of 10-year-old Québec and 10-11-year-old Jamaican study participants

Characteristic	Category	Québec	Jamaica	P-value
		% (n)	% (n)	
Sex	Girl	52.4 (624)	52.6 (881)	0.6792
	Boy	47.6 (566)	47.4 (793)	
Overweight or obese	No	74	89	<.0001
	Yes	26	11	
Family SES	Tertile 1 (Low)	33.0	41.3	<.0001
	Tertile 2 (Middle)	34.1	29.4	
	Tertile 3 (High)	32.9	29.3	
Household food insecurity	No	90.6	73.6	<.0001
	Yes	9.4	26.4	
Family type	Two-parent family	66.3	34.2	<.0001
	Blended family	17.0	29.7	
	Single-parent family	16.7	36.1	
Pastry consumption	Less than once a day	68.7	64.2	0.1375
	Once to less than twice a day	20.3	23.4	
	Twice a day or more	11.0	12.4	

TABLE 9.1   *(Continued)*

Characteristic	Category	Québec	Jamaica	P-value
		% (n)	% (n)	
Fruit consumption	Less than once a day	31.1	41.5	<.0001
	Once to less than twice a day	19.1	31.9	
	Twice a day or more	49.8	26.6	
Vegetable consumption	Less than once a day	27.1	59.0	<.0001
	Once to less than twice a day	18.8	25.3	
	Twice a day or more	57.1	15.7	
Physical activity (Québec)	Same, lower or much lower than other children	67.6	//////////	
	Higher or much higher than other children	32.4	//////////	
Physical activity (Jamaica)	None or low	//////////	51.9	
	Moderate or high	//////////	48.1	

Table 2 presents the prevalence of childhood overweight/obesity in Québec and Jamaica according to selected child, family, and household characteristics. In Québec, when boys and girls were analyzed together, the proportion of overweight/obese children was found to be higher in low-SES families (32.2%), in comparison to medium-SES (23.2%) or high-SES (22.2%) families. The proportion of overweight/obese children in food-insecure households (52.5%) was more than double the proportion in food-secure households (23.1%). A higher proportion of overweight/obesity was also observed in children from single-parent families and children who consumed vegetables less than once a day, in comparison to children living in other types of families and children who consumed vegetables more frequently per day, respectively (see also adjusted odds ratios in Table 3). While these trends were similar in boys and girls, the statistically significant findings indicated in Table 2 appear to be driven by differences observed among girls; no statistically significant differences were observed among boys.

In Jamaica, childhood overweight/obesity was significantly associated only with family SES and household food insecurity. The proportion of overweight/obese children was higher in high-SES families (13%) in comparison to medium-SES (12.2%) or low-SES (6.8%) families. Similarly, a higher proportion of overweight/obesity was found in children from food-secure households (12.1%) in comparison to those in food-insecure households (7.9%).

TABLE 9.2 Frequency of overweight or obesity in Québec and Jamaican children by selected characteristics, by sex and by both sexes combined.

Characteristic	Category	Overweight or obese Québec children			Overweight or obese Jamaican children		
		Girls	Boys	All	Girls	Boys	All
Sex	Girl	///////////	///////////	26.3	///////////	///////////	12.6
	Boy	///////////	///////////	25.3	///////////	///////////	9.2
Family SES	Tertile 1 (Low)	34.5*	29.6	32.2*	8.3	5.3*	6.8*
	Tertile 2 (Medium)	22.8	23.6	23.2	14.9	9.5	12.2
	Tertile 3 (High)	21.6	23.0	22.2	14.2	11.6	13.0
Household food insecurity	No	23.2*	23.1	23.1*	13.7	10.5	12.1*
	Yes	66.0	34.6	52.5	9.8	6.1	7.9
Family type	Two-parent family	21.7*	24.5	23.1*	13.8	10.8	12.5
	Blended family	28.8	27.0	28.1	13.5	8.7	11
	Single-parent family	41.9	27.6	35.2	10.8	8.2	9.5
Pastry consumption	Less than once a day	30.7*	25.6	28.4	13.5	10	11.9
	Once to less than twice a day	26.1	20.5	23.1	10.3	8.7	9.5
	Twice a day or more	10.4	24.9	17.1	9.2	6.7	7.9
Fruit consumption	Less than once a day	34.2	28.4	31.4	14.5	9.3	12
	Once to less than twice a day	26.9	19.1	22.8	10.9	9.9	10.4
	Twice a day or more	24.4	24.4	24.4	11.5	7.7	9.6
Vegetable	Less than once a day	41.9*	31.7	37.3*	13.1	9.1	11.2

TABLE 9.3 (Continued)

Characteristic	Category	Overweight or obese Québec children			Overweight or obese Jamaican children		
		Girls	Boys	All	Girls	Boys	All
consumption	Once to less than twice a day	19.9	22.7	21.2	12.5	9.4	10.9
	Twice a day or more	21.9	21.4	21.6	12.5	9.6	11.1
Physical activity (Québec)	Same, lower or much lower than other children	28.8	26.3	27.6	/////////////	/////////////	/////////////
	Higher or much higher than other children	20.4	23.4	21.8	/////////////	/////////////	/////////////
Physical activity (Jamaica)	None or low	/////////////	/////////////	/////////////	15.0*	9.1	12.5
	Moderate or high	/////////////	/////////////	/////////////	10.1	9.2	9.6

*Statistically significant association between the characteristic and the dependent variables within column (chi-square $P \leq 0.05$).

TABLE 9.3 Adjusted odds ratios (OR and 95% CI) for overweight and obese Québec and Jamaican children by selected characteristics, by sex and by both sexes combined

Characteristic	Category	Overweight or obese Québec children#			Overweight or obese Jamaican children##		
		Girls	Boys	All	Girls	Boys	All
Family SES	Tertile 1 (Low)	1	1	1	1	1	1
	Tertile 2 (Middle)	0.87 (0.5-1.5)	0.92 (0.5-1.6)	0.89 (0.6-1.3)	1.87 (1.0-3.4)*	1.75 (0.8-3.9)	1.83 (1.1-3.0)*
	Tertile 3 (High)	0.97 (0.5-1.7)	0.91 (0.5-1.7)	0.95 (0.6-1.4)	1.74 (0.9-3.3)	2.37 (1.2-4.9)*	2.00 (1.3-3.2)*
Family type	Two-parent family	1	1	1	1	1	1
	Blended family	0.91 (0.5-1.7)	1.14 (0.6-2.2)	1.0 (0.7-1.6)	1.0 (0.6-1.6)	0.59 (0.3-1.6)	0.82 (0.6-1.2)
	Single-parent family	1.82 (0.9-3.4)	1.37 (0.7-2.5)	1.63 (1.0-2.5)*	0.79 (0.4-1.3)	0.69 (0.3-1.2)	0.74 (0.5-1.1)
Household food insecurity	No	1	1	1	1	1	1
	Yes	4.99 (2.4-10.5)*	1.56 (0.7-3.3)	3.03 (1.8-5.0)*	0.72 (0.4-1.2)	0.58 (0.3-1.3)	0.65 (0.4-0.9)*

*Significantly different from the reference category ($P \leq 0.05$).
Models adjusted for consumption of pastry and vegetables and for physical activity.
Models adjusted for physical activity.

Sex-specific analyses yielded several significant associations in both the Québec and Jamaican samples. For girls in Québec, childhood overweight/ obesity was significantly associated with family SES, household food insecurity, family type, daily consumption of pastries, and daily consumption of vegetables. For boys, no association was observed between childhood overweight/obesity and any of the child, family, or household variables examined. In Jamaica, when the data were analyzed separately for girls and boys, only level of physical activity showed a significant association with overweight/obesity in girls, and only family SES was associated with overweight/obesity in boys.

Multivariate analyses (Table 3) revealed that children in food-insecure households in Québec had odds of 3.03 (95% CI 1.8-5.0) for being overweight or obese, with odds of 4.99 (95% CI 2.4-10.5) for being overweight or obese specifically in girls (when analyzed by gender) in comparison to children in food-secure households. Single-parenting also increased the odds of being overweight or obese by 63% in Québec children. Family SES was no longer significant in multivariate analyses. In Jamaica, the association with childhood overweight/ obesity was reversed: higher SES was associated with increased overweight/ obesity, and food insecurity was associated with reduced overweight/obesity. More specifically, Jamaican children in food-insecure households had odds of 0.65 (95% CI 0.4-0.9) for being overweight or obese in comparison to those in food-secure households. Similarly, Jamaican children in middle SES (OR 1.83, 95% CI 1.1-3.0) and high SES (OR 2.00, 95% CI 1.3-3.2) families had increased odds of being overweight or obese in comparison to children in low SES families. When boys and girls were considered separately, only SES remained positively associated with overweight/obesity. In comparison to boys and girls in low SES families, boys from high-SES families had odds of 2.37 (95% CI 1.2-4.9) for being overweight or obese, and girls from middle-SES families had odds of 1.87 (95% CI 1.0-3.4). Odds ratio point estimates for boys from middle-SES families and girls from high-SES families increased but failed to reach statistical significance.

9.4 DISCUSSION

The aims of this study were twofold. First, we sought to determine whether household food insecurity was significantly related to childhood overweight/ obesity in Québec and in Jamaica. Second, we explored possible gender differences in these associations.

9.4.1   Overweight and Obesity

Overall we found that the prevalence of overweight/obesity differed considerably between Québec (26%) and Jamaica (11%). Findings from the Québec sample corresponded to estimates for Canada as a whole [28] and were also comparable to estimates from other developed countries, such as the United States [52]. However, the prevalence of overweight/obesity among Jamaican children appeared lower than previously reported for similarly aged children [29]. The estimates obtained in the aforementioned study was, however, confined to the urban area of Kingston; whereas, data for our study were representative of all 14 parishes in Jamaica. The use of universal cut-points for overweight/obesity in both adults and children is somewhat controversial due to differences in race/ethnicity and the effects of maturation and genetics [53–55]. Our findings showed clearly that obesity is a critical health problem in both countries. The large disparity in the prevalence of overweight/obesity observed may be attributable to genetic, psychosocial, economic, dietary, and other environmental or behavioral factors, such as physical activity [53]. The disparity may also reflect differences in how the economies of these two countries are integrated into the global economy. In rural areas of developing countries, individuals may have less access to low-nutrient, energy-dense products that are high in sugar and fat, and indeed underweight can be more prevalent than overweight/obesity [14, 56].

9.4.2   Household Food Insecurity

The prevalence of food insecurity among children in Québec (9.4%) was slightly higher than the one reported for the province of Québec through the 2008 Canadian Community Health Survey [30, 57]. In 2008, 14.6% of households in the United States reported food insecurity; however, it was not clear how many of these households included children [58]. The present study estimates household food insecurity among Jamaican children to be at a prevalence of 26.4%; to our knowledge, these findings are the first to provide such an estimate. This percentage is disproportionately lower than estimates reported for other developing countries, including an urban population in Caracas, Venezuela (64%) [59], urban and rural samples from Bolivia (70%) [60], and school children 5-12 years old in Bogota, Columbia (76%) [61].

9.4.3   Association between Household food Insecurity and Overweight/Obesity

The present report confirms our hypothesis indicating that in Québec, children who live in food-insecure households have higher odds of being overweight or obese in comparison to children who live in food-secure households. By contrast, in Jamaica food insecurity was associated with decreased odds of being overweight or obese. Similarly, recent studies in Canada and the United States have reported a positive association between food insecurity and childhood obesity [20–22]. However, other studies conducted in similar contexts (e.g., the United States and Mexico) reported negative [23–25] or no relationships between food insecurity and childhood obesity [26, 27, 62]. As Gundersen and colleagues (2008) suggested, these inconsistencies may be explained by differences in the way food insecurity was measured. For example, in a developing country like Trinidad, Gulliford (2003) showed that food insecurity was associated with an increased likelihood of underweight and not obesity among adults [63]. Unfortunately, studies that might shed light on the relationship between food insecurity and overweight/obesity in children are scarce in developing countries.

One possible explanation for disparities in the relationship between food insecurity and overweight/obesity between developed and developing middle-income countries is that the food-insecurity and overweight/obesity pathways may be different. For example, in developed countries like Canada, social support services available to low-income and food-insecure families (e.g., food subsidies, food stamps, social assistance) have been associated with increased overweight/obesity [64, 65]. This may be due to an increased consumption of cheaper and refined carbohydrates, sweetened beverages, high-fat meats, and lower consumption of fruits and vegetables because of monetary constraints. It is known that poorer families may substitute higher-quality foods for cheaper, lower-quality foods and this practice has been associated with overweight and obesity in developed countries [66–68].

By contrast, developing countries like Jamaica have limited social support systems to help with food subsidies. As a result, children from food-insecure and poorer families consume fewer total calories and so are less likely to be overweight or obese. Moreover, the present study's findings may explain why food insecurity and SES share a pathway in relation to overweight and obesity in both countries. Unlike the association between SES and overweight/obesity in Jamaica, the prevalence of overweight/obesity was higher among children from low-SES families and/or children from single-parent families in Québec.

In multivariate analyses, SES did not prove to be a significant factor, probably due to the inadequate sample size and its attendant inability to show statistical significance. By contrast, in Jamaica, both variables remained significant, thereby associating high SES with overweight/obesity, whereas food insecurity was associated with reduced odds of overweight/obesity.

9.4.4   Gender Differences

In Québec, when boys and girls were considered separately, food insecurity significantly associated with being overweight or obese only in girls. In children from food-insecure households in Québec, disproportionately more girls were overweight or obese than boys. Additionally, among children who were overweight, more girls than boys (41.9% vs. 27.6%) had single-parent families, and more girls than boys came from low-SES families (34.5% vs. 29.6%). These findings show that the majority of girls and boys from food-insecure households lived in two very different family environments. This difference may explain the gender-specific relationship between household food insecurity and childhood overweight/obesity observed in our study. Moreover, given that, in almost all cases (99%), the head of single-parent families were women in the Québec sample [69], perhaps having an overweight/obese mother exerted a strong influence on girls' body weights since modeling effectively transmits values, beliefs, and practices [70]; however this explanation requires further investigation. When the time and desire to cook are limited among single mothers, they may resort to buying inexpensive, energy-dense, processed foods that have been associated with the obesity epidemic [67].

On the other hand, in Jamaica the prevalence of overweight/obesity was higher among children living in two-parent and blended families, although group differences were not significant at the univariate or multivariate levels. Additionally, boys from higher SES families had greater odds of being overweight/obese than did girls. A positive association between higher SES and overweight/obesity among men, women, and children has been reported in the literature on developing countries [16, 17]. Among Jamaican children, the food insecurity-overweight/obesity relationship yielded similar results when boys and girls were analyzed separately. This result has been previously reported for adults in other developing countries [63].

The gender-based differences observed in the present study among children from Québec have been previously reported for adults in other developed countries, such that women in food-insecure households were found to have a higher prevalence of overweight/obesity in comparison to men [45, 65, 71]. Few studies have examined gender differences in the association between food insecurity and overweight/obesity in children. Two studies found that food-insecure girls were more likely to be overweight than their food-secure counterparts; whereas, among boys, there were no significant findings [22, 41]. In developing countries like Jamaica, these previously unstudied emergent differences may well be attributable to the status of the nutritional and epidemiological transition [72, 73]. Other mitigating factors, such as family type and SES which our study shows to be present in both developed and developing countries, are consistent with those reported in the literature [16, 17, 64].

9.4.5 Strengths and Limitations

The most notable strength of this study is that both samples were statistically representative of their populations and both employed standardized weights. The response rate was greater than or equal to 85% in both samples. The Jamaican sample size was adjusted for a 10% refusal rate. The results of the study can thus be generalized to other cases. In addition, objective anthropometric measures of body mass index were obtained.

As our study explores the relationship between food insecurity and overweight/obesity in children from both a developed and a developing country, certain limitations exist. First, given the cross-sectional nature of the data, causality cannot be assigned to the associations observed in this study. Elucidating these relationships will require retrospective longitudinal studies that make it possible to examine temporal sequences of events [41]. Issues relating to the measurement of food insecurity also did not allow us to examine the effects of different levels of food insecurity on overweight/obesity. Furthermore, in the Québec sample, children's level of physical activity was parent-reported rather than measured; thus, children were classified according to subjective information. A number of studies have shown that parents have difficulty accurately estimating and recalling their children's physical activity patterns (e.g., type, intensity, duration, frequency) [34]. Finally, the derivation of the SES variable in the Jamaican sample did not include conventional indicators, such as income and education, as they were not available. This may have resulted in a SES index with reduced discriminatory capacity.

9.5 CONCLUSIONS

Food insecurity appears to be positively associated with childhood overweight/ obesity in children from the province of Québec, Canada. An inverse relationship is observed among children in Jamaica, a developing country. Gender differences are also apparent in the food insecurity-childhood overweight/obesity association in Québec, such that significantly more girls are found to be "at risk" in comparison to boys. Sex differences in the association between SES, family type, and childhood overweight/obesity are observed in both Québec and Jamaica. The findings of this study suggest that public health interventions which aim to stem the epidemic of overweight/obesity should look beyond biology and individual behaviours to the root causes of the epidemic. Family dynamics, gender differences, and trends in the global food system all influence the spread of overweight/obesity, both in developed and developing countries.

REFERENCES

1. Wang Y, Lobstein T: Worldwide trends in childhood overweight and obesity. Int J Pediatr Obes 2006, 1:11–25.
2. Rokholm B, Baker JL, Sorensen TIA: The levelling off of the obesity epidemic since the year 1999 - a review of evidence and perspectives. Obes Rev 2010, 11:835–846.
3. Ball GDC, McCargar LJ: Childhood obesity in Canada: A review of prevalence estimates and risk factors for cardiovascular diseases and type 2 diabetes. Can J Appl Physiol 2003, 28:117–140.
4. Daniels SR: The consequences of childhood overweight and obesity. Future Child 2006, 16:47–67.
5. Reilly JJ, Methven E, McDowell ZC, Hacking B, Alexander D, Stewart L, Kelnar CJH: Health consequences of obesity. Arch Dis Child 2003, 88:748–752.
6. Slyper AH: The pediatric obesity epidemic: Causes and controversies. J Clin Endocrinol Metab 2004, 89:2540–2547.
7. Francis DK, Van den Broeck J, Younger N, McFarlane S, Rudder K, Gordon-Strachan G, Grant A, Johnson A, Tulloch-Reid M, Wilks R: Fast-food and sweetened beverage consumption: association with overweight and high waist circumference in adolescents. Public Health Nutr 2009, 12:1106–1114.
8. Harnack LJ, Jeffery RW, Boutelle KN: Temporal trends in energy intake in the United States: an ecologic perspective. Am J Clin Nutr 2000, 71:1478–1484.
9. Kant AK, Graubard BI: Energy density of diets reported by American adults: association with food group intake, nutrient intake, and body weight. Int J Obes 2005, 29:950–956.
10. Nicklas TA, Elkasabany A, Srinivasan SR, Berenson G: Trends in nutrient intake of 10-year-old children over two decades (1973–1994) The Bogalusa Heart Study. Am J Epidemiol 2001, 153:969–977.

11. Troiano RP, Briefel RR, Carroll MD, Bialostosky K: Energy and fat intakes of children and adolescents in the United States: data from the National Health and Nutrition Examination Surveys. Am J Clin Nutr 2000, 72:1343S-1353S.

12. Doak CM, Adair LS, Bentley M, Monteiro C, Popkin BM: The dual burden household and the nutrition transition paradox. Int J Obes 2005, 29:129-136.

13. Wang YF, Monteiro C, Popkin BM: Trends of obesity and underweight in older children and adolescents in the United States, Brazil, China, and Russia. Am J Clin Nutr 2002, 75:971-977.

14. Kosti RI, Panagiotakos DB: The epidemic of obesity in children and adolescents in the world. Cent Eur J Public Health 2006, 14:151-159.

15. Shrewsbury V, Wardle J: Socioeconomic status and adiposity in childhood: A systematic review of cross-sectional studies 1990-2005. Obesity (Silver Spring) 2008, 16:275-284.

16. McLaren L: Socioeconomic status and obesity. Epidemiol Rev 2007, 29:29-48.

17. Sobal J, Stunkard AJ: Socioeconomic-Status and Obesity - A Review of the Literature. Psychol Bull 1989, 105:260-275.

18. Mendez MA, Monteiro CA, Popkin BM: Overweight exceeds underweight among women in most developing countries. Am J Clin Nutr 2005, 81:714-721.

19. Food and Agriculture Organization (FAO): Food Security. Rome: FAO; 2006.

20. Casey PH, Simpson PM, Gossett JM, Bogle ML, Champagne CM, Connell C, Harsha D, McCabe-Sellers B, Robbins JM, Stuff JE: The association of child and household food insecurity with childhood overweight status. Pediatrics 2006, 118:E1406-E1413.

21. Dubois L, Farmer A, Girard M, Porcherie M: Family food insufficiency is related to overweight among preschoolers. Soc Sci Med 2006, 63:1503-1516.

22. Jyoti DF, Frongillo EA, Jones SJ: Food insecurity affects school children's academic performance, weight gain, and social skills. J Nutr 2005, 135:2831-2839.

23. Jimenez-Cruz A, Bacardi-Gascon M, Spindler AA: Obesity and hunger among Mexican-Indian migrant children on the US-Mexico border. Int J Obes 2003, 27:740-747.

24. Matheson DM, Varady J, Varady A, Killen JD: Household food security and nutritional status of Hispanic children in the fifth grade. Am J Clin Nutr 2002, 76:210-217.

25. Rose D, Bodor JN: Household food insecurity and overweight status in young school children: Results from the Early Childhood Longitudinal Study. Pediatrics 2006, 117:464-473.

26. Gundersen C, Lohman BJ, Eisenmann JC, Garasky S, Stewart SD: Child-specific food insecurity and overweight are not associated in a sample of 10- to 15-year-old low-income youth. J Nutr 2008, 138:371-378.

27. Kaiser LL, Melgar-Quinonez HR, Lamp CL, John MC, Sutherlin JM, Harwood JO: Food security and nutritional outcomes of preschool-age Mexican-American children. J Am Diet Assoc 2002, 102:924-929.

28. Shields M: Measured obesity: overweight Canadian children and adolescents in Nutrition: Findings from the Canadian Community Health survey. Ottawa: Statistics Canada; 2009.

29. Jackson M, Samms-Vaughan M, Ashley D: Nutritional status of 11-12-year-old Jamaican children: coexistence of under- and overnutrition in early adolescence. Public Health Nutr 2002, 5:281-288.

30. Canada Health: Canadian Community Health Survey. Ottawa: Health Canada; 2008.

31. Dubois L, Bédard B, Girard M, Beauchesne E: L'alimentation. Etude longitudinale du développement des enfants du Québec (ELDEQ 1998-2002). Les nourrissons de 5 mois. Québec: Institut de la statistique du Québec 2000.

32. Fox K, Gordon-Strachan G: Jamaican Youth Risk and Resiliency Behaviour Survey 2005. 2007.
33. Planning Institute of Jamaica: Planning Institute of Jamaica, Economic and Social Survey of Jamaica. Planning Institute of Jamaica: Kingston; 2004.
34. Goran MI: Measurement issues related to studies of childhood obesity: Assessment of body composition, body fat distribution, physical activity, and food intake. Pediatrics 1998, 101:505–518.
35. Statistical Institute of Jamaica (STATIN): Demographic Statistics (2001). Kingston: STATIN; 2001.
36. Global Tobacco Surveillance System Collaborating Group: Global Tobacco Surveillance System (GTSS): purpose, production, and potential. J Sch Health 2005, 75:15–24.
37. Desrosiers H, Dubois L, Beal Bédard: Enquête de nutrition auprès des enfants québecois de 4 ans. Québec: Institut de la Statistique du Québec 2005.
38. Cole TJ, Bellizzi MC, Flegal KM, Dietz WH: Establishing a standard definition for child overweight and obesity worldwide: international survey. Br Med J 2000, 320:1240–1243.
39. Canada Health: Canadian Community Health Survey Cycle 2.2, Nutrition Income-Related Household Food Security in Canada. Ottawa: Health Canada; 2004.
40. Anderson SA: Core Indicators of Nutritional State for Difficult-To-Sample Populations. J Nutr 1990, 120:1559–1599.
41. Alaimo K, Olson CM, Frongillo EA: Low family income and food insufficiency in relation to overweight in US children - Is there a paradox? Arch Pediatr Adolesc Med 2001, 155:1161–1167.
42. Rose D, Gundersen C, Oliveira V: Socio-economic determinant of food insecurity in the United States: Evidence from the SIPP and CSF II datasets. Washington, DC: US Department of Agriculture; 1998.
43. Briefel RR, Woteki CE: Development of Food Sufficiency Questions for the 3Rd National-Health and Nutrition Examination Survey. J Nutr Educ 1992, 24:S24-S28.
44. Carlson S, Briefel RR: The USDA and NHANES food insufficiency question as an indicator of hunger and food insecurity. In Conference on food security measurement and research: Papers and proceedings. Alexandria, VA: US Department of Agriculture, Food and Consumer Services; 1995.
45. Basiotis PP: Validity of the self-reported food insufficiency status item in the US Department of Agriculture Food Consumption Surveys. In Proceedings of the 1992 annual meeting of the American council in the consumer interest, March 25–28. Toronto, ON; 1992.
46. Cristofar SP, Basiotis PP: Dietary Intakes and Selected Characteristics of Women Ages 19–50 Years and Their Children Ages 1–5 Years by Reported Perception of Food Sufficiency. J Nutr Educ 1992, 24:53–58.
47. Pan American Health Organization: The Caribbean Youth Survey 1997. 1997.
48. Craig CL, Marshall AL, Sjostrom M, Bauman AE, Booth ML, Ainsworth BE, Pratt M, Ekelund U, Yngve A, Sallis JF, Oja P: International physical activity questionnaire: 12-country reliability and validity. Med Sci Sports and Exerc 2003, 35:1381–1395.
49. Jetté M, Des Groseilliers L: Survey description and methodology in Longitudinal Study of Child Development in Québec (ELDEQ 1998–2002) (Vol. 1, 1). Québec: Institut de la statistique du Québec; 2000.
50. Willms JD, Shields M: A measure of socioeconomic status for the National Longitudinal Study of Children. Report prepared for Statistics Canada 1996.

51. Cox B, Cohen S: Methodological Issues jor Health Care Surveys. New York: Dekker; 1985.
52. Hedley AA, Ogden CL, Johnson CL, Carroll MD, Curtin LR, Flegal KM: Prevalence of overweight and obesity among US children, adolescents, and adults, 1999–2002. J Am Med Assoc 2004, 291:2847–2850.
53. Bray GA: In defense of a body mass index of 25 as the cut-off point for defining overweight. Obes Res 1998, 6:461–462.
54. Deurenberg P, Yap M, van Staveren WA: Body mass index and percent body fat: a meta-analysis among different ethnic groups. Int J Obes 1998, 22:1164–1171.
55. World Health Organization: The Asia-Pacific Perspective: Redefining Obesity and its Treatment. Sydney: Health Communications; 2000.
56. Sobal J: Commentary: Globalization and the epidemiology of obesity. Int J Epidemiol 2001, 30:1136–1137.
57. Health Canada: Canadian Community Health Survey Cycle 2.2 Nutrition Income-Related Household Food Security in Canada. Ottawa: Health Canada; 2004.
58. Nord M, Andrews M, Carlson S: Household Food Security in the United States, 2008. 2009.
59. Lorenzana PA, Mercado C: Measuring household food security in poor Venezuelan households. Public Health Nutr 2002, 5:851–857.
60. Melgar-Quinonez HR, Zubieta AC, MkNelly B, Nteziyaremye A, Gerardo MFD, Dunford C: Household food insecurity and food expenditure in Bolivia, Burkina Faso, and the Philippines. J Nutr 2006, 136:1431–1437.
61. Isanaka S, Mora-Plazas M, Lopez-Arana S, Baylin A, Villamor E: Food insecurity is highly prevalent and predicts underweight but not overweight in adults and school children from Bogota, Colombia. J Nutr 2007, 137:2747–2755.
62. Gundersen C, Garasky S, Lohman BJ: Food Insecurity Is Not Associated with Childhood Obesity as Assessed Using Multiple Measures of Obesity. J Nutr 2009, 139:1173–1178.
63. Gulliford MC, Mahabir D, Rocke B: Food insecurity, food choices, and body mass index in adults: nutrition transition in Trinidad and Tobago. Int J Epidemiol 2003, 32:508–516.
64. Gibson LY, Byrne SM, Davis EA, Blair E, Jacoby P, Zubrick SR: The role of family and maternal factors in childhood obesity. Med J Aust 2007, 186:591–595.
65. Townsend MS, Peerson J, Love B, Achterberg C, Murphy SP: Food insecurity is positively related to overweight in women. J Nutr 2001, 131:1738–1745.
66. Dietz WH: Does Hunger Cause Obesity. Pediatrics 1995, 95:766–767.
67. Drewnowski A, Specter SE: Poverty and obesity: the role of energy density and energy costs. Am J Clin Nutr 2004, 79:6–16.
68. Wilde PE, Peterman JN: Individual weight change is associated with household food security status. J Nutr 2006, 136:1395–1400.
69. Institut de la Statistique du Québec: Family, child care and Neighbourhood characteristics. Québec; 2000.
70. Maccoby EE: Social Development. In Psychological Growth and the Parent-Child Relationship. New York: Harcourt Brace Janovich; 1980.
71. Olson CM: Nutrition and health outcomes associated with food insecurity and hunger. J Nutr 1999, 129:521S-524S.
72. Gulliford MC: Epidemiological transition in Trinidad and Tobago, West Indies 1953–1992. Int J Epidemiol 1996, 25:357–365.
73. Wilks R, Bennett F, Forrester T, McFarlane-Anderson N: Chronic diseases: the new epidemic. West Indian Med J 1998,47(4):40–44.

Community Perspectives on Food Insecurity and Obesity: Focus Groups with Caregivers of Métis and Off-Reserve First Nations Children

Jasmin Bhawra, Martin J. Cooke, Rhona Hanning, Piotr Wilk, and Shelley L. H. Gonneville

10.1 DILAPIDATED DWELLING

Child obesity is an urgent public health issue in Canada and other wealthy countries. The World Health Organization defines obesity as the accumulation of excess fat to the point where it has adverse impacts on health [1]. Approximately one third of Canadian children between the ages of 5 to 17 years could be considered overweight or obese, with some populations at an even higher risk [2]. Aboriginal children are disproportionately affected by obesity, as they are twice as likely to be classified as obese compared to their non-Aboriginal Canadian counterparts [3, 4]. This is true for children of each of the three Aboriginal groups identified in the 1982 *Constitution Act*—First Nations, Métis and Inuit—which together make up about four per cent of the Canadian population or 1.5 million people [5], and for those living in urban areas as well as in rural or remote First Nations or Inuit communities. Although obtaining a comparable measurement of child obesity among Aboriginal children can be problematic, an estimated 20 % of First Nations children living off reserve[1] (aged 5 to 17), and 16.9 % of Métis children could be classified as obese [4], compared with 11.7 % of Canadian children aged 5 to 17 [2].

The poorer average health of Aboriginal peoples, relative to other citizens in wealthy former colonies including Canada, the United States, Australia and New Zealand [6], as well as poorer ones in South and Central America and elsewhere in the "new world" has been well documented [7]. Although colonization progressed differently in these countries and the colonists differed somewhat in their orientations to Aboriginal peoples, including in the degree of violence employed in subjugating them, the overarching logic of colonialism was the same. This included dispossession from traditional lands and waters, devaluation of indigenous languages and cultures, and attempts either to assimilate dominated people to settler economic systems or to relegate them to marginal "reserve" lands [8].

In Canada, the mechanisms of colonialism have included the *Indian Act*, which continues to legally define and fragment Aboriginal peoples, and residential schooling, which led to generations of Aboriginal children being raised in institutions and away from their families [8]. Colonial institutions and practices have had different implications for each of the three recognized Aboriginal groups in Canada. "First Nations," an umbrella term referring to about a dozen major linguistic and cultural groups living across the continent below the Arctic, have been the subjects of the *Indian Act* and reserve system, resulting in a situation in which about half of those identifying as First Nations are legally Registered Indians, with roughly 60 % of those living in First Nations reserves. Somewhat paradoxically, Métis have suffered from not being recognized as an Aboriginal people. The result of a historical blending of European and First Nations cultures, mainly around the fur trade in Western Canada, Métis ethnogenesis and the development of a distinct culture and language have been identified as occurring before Canadian confederation in 1867 [9]. For most of their history, Métis were recognized neither as an Aboriginal people nor as fully European/Canadian, resulting in exclusion from treaties and land settlements and, until recently, from Aboriginal hunting and gathering rights. Inuit, the people of the North, were the last to be fully colonized. After the Second World War, the federal government pursued an active program of assimilation of Inuit [10], and in recent decades economic activity around resource development in the North have further contributed to many Inuit finding themselves culturally and economically dislocated, neither able to practice a traditional way of life nor integrated into a modern wage economy.

The results of historical and contemporary colonial practices can be seen today in ongoing disparities in income, educational attainment and labour force participation, each of which are considered important "upstream" determinants of population health [11]. Although the income gaps narrowed somewhat in the 1990s, First Nations Inuit and Métis continue to have significantly lower average incomes than non-Aboriginal Canadians, and this is true for the more than half of the population that currently lives in cities[2], as well as those who live in First Nations reserves or Inuit communities [12].

The relationships between income inequalities, other social determinants, and particular health outcomes are complex, and may involve material standards of living, psychosocial effects, social capital, and other pathways [13]. In the particular case of obesity among Aboriginal children, Willows Hanley and Delormier (2012) have proposed a socioecological framework to understanding these effects [14]. At the most proximate level, children's weights are affected by their energy intake and expenditure, mediated by genetic factors. However, children's diets and physical activities are themselves shaped by family characteristics, including incomes, knowledge about healthy eating and exercise, and parents' behaviours. These are further affected by factors associated with neighbourhood and communities, such as access to safe play spaces and the local cost of food, or the availability of recreation programs. All of these can be placed within the context of macro-level social and economic structures, including the industrial production of food and the wage economy. Critically, in the case of Aboriginal peoples, this macro context includes colonialism and continued social and economic marginalization [14].

The research reported in this paper is part of a broader project to understand some of the specific mechanisms that produce the excess risk of obesity among Aboriginal children to inform the design of public health interventions to reduce this risk. In this paper we focus on the role of "food security" in this respect. Aboriginal peoples in Canada are at a higher risk for food insecurity, generally defined as the limited or uncertain availability of nutritionally adequate and safe foods [15, 16, 17]. This is most obviously the case for rural and remote First Nations reserves and Inuit communities, in which the high cost of fresh foods transported from the south has combined with decreasing use of traditional food sources to result in diets characterised by consumption of inexpensive, but nutritionally poor, packaged foods [18, 19]. However, urban First Nations and Métis, who have not been part of the reserve system, have higher risk for food insecurity as well as for obesity. Aboriginal households in urban areas, and also in non-remote rural areas, have a risk of food insecurity that is up to three times that of non-Aboriginal households [8, 17].

Much of this higher prevalence of both food insecurity and obesity is certainly due to higher rates of poverty among Aboriginal peoples [20]. Lower household income has been found to be related to a higher risk of obesity among Métis children [21], and neighbourhood income has been related to child obesity among Canadian children in general [22]. The specific mechanisms that connect food insecurity and child obesity are not necessarily obvious, though, nor are the options for addressing these issues. Among low-income Canadians in general, nutritional knowledge and food skills have been suggested as possible factors connecting income to nutrition, although the evidence indicates that these effects might not be significant [23], and that it is income adequacy that is the critical factor [24]. When considering the nutrition of children, mothers' strategies for mitigating the effects of food insecurity may include reducing their own consumption, in addition to the use of food banks, community gardens, and community kitchens [25]. There is evidence, however, that those community-based services are under-utilized by the food insecure and are therefore not reaching the intended populations [26].

In the case of Aboriginal populations, the connections are even less clear. A central consideration in the definition of food insecurity should be the cultural appropriateness and acceptability of available food, not just its affordability [27]. For Métis and First Nations people in urban areas, the experience of food insecurity, food preferences, coping strategies, and the perceived connections between the food environment and children's health may be different from those of non-Aboriginal Canadians or from those living in discrete Aboriginal communities. Appropriate strategies for addressing these issues may also be different, and should not simply be extrapolated from other contexts.

This study helps to address the lack of previous qualitative research on food insecurity and obesity among Métis and urban First Nations children. It was conducted in the context of a broader mixed-methods study of the determinants of child obesity among Aboriginal children, with the intention of identifying promising directions for community-based programming to reduce obesity risk3. Using semi-structured focus groups with parents and caregivers of Métis and First Nations children, we explored parents' perceptions of the factors that affected the ability of families to provide culturally appropriate and healthful food, and the strategies that community members used to address food insecurity. We draw conclusions regarding the connections between food insecurity and child obesity in this population, and propose some avenues for further research.

10.2 METHODS

10.2.1 Study Design

A total of four focus groups were conducted with First Nations and Métis care-givers in London and Midland-Penetanguishene, respectively. Two focus groups were held in Midland-Penetanguishene in partnership with the Métis Nation of Ontario, and the latter two focus groups took place in London in collaboration with a local Aboriginal health centre. These locations were chosen because they are urban settings with relatively large First Nations and Métis populations, but represent different geographic contexts.

London is a medium-sized Canadian city located in southwestern Ontario with a population of 467,225 people in 2011 [28]. It is located close to several First Nations reserves and is approximately halfway between Toronto, Ontario and Detroit, Michigan. According to the 2011 National Household Survey, 6200 people living in the city identified themselves as First Nations, and approximately 2000 as Métis [28] (Fig. 1).

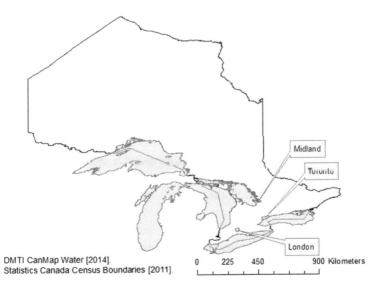

DMTI CanMap Water [2014].
Statistics Canada Census Boundaries [2011].

0   225   450   900 Kilometers

FIGURE 10.1   Location of London and Midland, Ontario.

Midland-Penetanguishene, which includes the Town of Midland and several nearby townships, is a more rural community located in Northern Ontario with a total population of approximately 43,000 people in 2011 [29, 30]. It experiences seasonal tourism, which brings upwards of 100,000 visitors in the summer months. Métis people are 11 % of the population (4800 people) in Midland-Penetanguishene making it a major concentration of Métis in the province. Approximately 1500 residents identified themselves as First Nations in the 2011 National Household Survey [29, 30].

Purposive, convenience sampling was used in collaboration with local Aboriginal partner organizations. Recruitment was conducted using advertisements in local newspapers as well as direct referrals by collaborating organizations. The convenience sampling method was appropriate for this group, as existing rapport and trust were important to ensuring that potential respondents felt comfortable sharing their insights with our research group. Parents or caregivers of Métis or First Nations children under 18 were invited to participate in the focus group sessions. The recruitment referred to "parents and caregivers", as opposed to only parents, because Aboriginal children are more likely to live in intergenerational households and parents may not be the primary guardians [31, 32], and we therefore use "caregivers" in the remainder of the paper. Income level, food security, and child weight status were not used as inclusion criteria in order to capture the broad range of respondents' experiences, promote inclusivity, and because of the sensitive nature of the topics discussed.

10.2.2 Participants and Procedure

A total of 32 caregivers were interviewed during the 90-minute sessions, with each focus group ranging from 5 to 11 participants. As suggested by collaborating organizations, the discussions were opened by an Elder or spiritual leader, who remained present for the session to offer support should any difficult or upsetting issues be brought up. All sessions were led by the same experienced Indigenous facilitator. The interview guide and focus group procedure were reviewed and approved by the research ethics boards at the University of Waterloo and Western University.

The focus groups were held in July 2011 and December 2011 in Midland-Penetanguishene, and December 2012 and March 2013 in London, Ontario. Information and consent forms were administered prior to the focus groups, and background questionnaires were completed following the focus groups to obtain basic demographic information and provide an opportunity for additional feedback.

The interview guide included questions about the health of children in the community, as well as barriers and facilitators to healthy eating and physical activity. Questions were kept open ended and phrased to capture community-level issues and examples, however the majority of participants drew from personal experiences during the discussions.

10.2.3   Data Analysis and Qualitative Rigor

All focus groups were audio recorded and professionally transcribed. Participants' identities were concealed throughout the data analysis and care was taken to ensure that identities could not be revealed in the quotations selected for reporting results. Participants were given the option to withdraw from the focus groups at any time. A thematic analysis was conducted involving coding individual transcripts into major themes using NVivo qualitative data analysis software Version 10 (2013) [33]. Codes were created for distinct ideas or concepts and organized into a coding manual. Transcripts were then uploaded into NVivo, and codes from the manual were entered as nodes into the program. This process allowed for reoccurring, prominent themes to be identified and examined within and across focus groups.

Experiences with food insecurity, coping strategies, as well as barriers and facilitators to healthy eating were themes of particular interest. While the coding manual was initially organized based on a priori research questions and concepts, including the barriers and facilitators to healthy eating, the content of the coding manual was modified as the analyses proceeded, and the research questions provided a general focus for conducting the analysis instead of a specific set of expectations or findings.

The next step involved testing the reliability and dependability of these codes to ensure rigor in this qualitative study. A reliability check was conducted using second coders. After the initial coding and coding manual development, two additional coders were provided with a copy of the coding manual and asked to re-code all transcripts. If a code was missing or inappropriately assigned, the second coders modified the manual accordingly. After debriefing with the second coders, a consensus was reached on all codes, which were then entered into NVivo. Dependability of the results was calculated using inter-rater reliability. The inter-rater reliability between the first and second coders was 88 % for the focus groups in Midland-Penetanguishene and 85 % in London, which surpasses the minimum requirement of 70 % suggested by Miles and Huberman (1994) [34]. Following the data analysis, reports were produced for the collaborating Métis and First Nations organizations to ensure the applicability of the findings and appropriateness of interpretation.

10.3   RESULTS

Twenty-three caregivers of Métis children and nine caregivers of First Nations children participated in the focus group discussions. The majority of respondents were women (81 %). Demographic characteristics from the two focus groups can be found in Tables 1 and 2.

TABLE 10.1   Demographic Characteristics of First Nations Caregivers from Focus Groups in London, Ontario

	Number	Percent
Gender		
Male	1	11 %
Female	8	89 %
Total participants	9	100 %
Years lived in the community		
Less than 1	0	0 %
1 to 5	2	22 %
6 to 10	1	11 %
11 to 19	1	11 %
20 to 25	1	11 %
30 to 34	2	22 %
35 to 39	0	0 %
40 +	1	11 %
Total Participants	8a	100 %

The thematic analysis of respondents' statements provided detailed insight into community members' challenges with healthy eating and coping strategies. Two key barriers to children's healthy diets that were raised by respondents were low income and difficulty in physically accessing fresh foods. It is important to note that the facilitators did not present income inadequacy and food insecurity as topics, rather they were brought up by participants as key factors which

TABLE 10.2 Demographic Characteristics of Métis Caregivers from Focus Groups in Midland-Penetanguishine, Ontario

	Number	Percent		Number	Percent
Gender			Number of children in the household		
Male	5	22 %	One	6	30 %
Female	18	78 %	Two	5	25 %
Total	23	100 %	Three	3	15 %
Years lived in the community			None/no response	6	30 %
Less than 1	2	9%	Total Households	20	100 %
1 to 5	2	9%			
6 to 10	2	9%	Ages of children in the household		
11 to 20	2	9%	1 to 4	5	19 %
20 to 25	2	9%	5 to 9	3	12 %
30 to 34	6	26 %	10 to 13	5	19 %
35 to 39	2	9%	14 to 16	7	27 %
40 +	5	22 %	17 to 23	6	23 %
Total Participants	23	100 %	Total children	26	100 %

affected Aboriginal parents' ability to provide nutritious food for their families. The availability of traditional foods was also raised as a concern. Participants also discussed various coping strategies for dealing with food insecurity, and identified ways that these strategies might be leading to the risk of obesity among Aboriginal children. These main themes are described briefly below.

10.3.1   Low Income as a Main Determinant

A majority of participants felt that the unaffordability of healthy food was an overarching barrier to improving children's diets. Several caregivers regarded healthy food options to be too costly, especially as compared to processed or convenience foods that were at a lower cost. A caregiver from Midland-Penetanguishene said:

> So, you know, the fattier foods are the lowest price and they go a lot further. So, you're going to see obesity in that stereotypical low-income/one income family. And if you take a two-income family, yes, you know what, there's more money coming in. So, yes, they can get the fresh fruits, they can get the fresh vegetables, they can buy the milk, they can, you know, they don't have to live on Kraft Dinner and soup.

For some families, the issue was not necessarily the cost of healthy food in particular, but rather that food in general was unaffordable. However, some respondents indicated that families who could afford more healthy food might still consume "junk" food. A First Nations caregiver stated:

> So yeah, it depends on the parents, if they're working they can afford more food for their kids and then they buy both food, like the health food and the junk food at the same time.

10.3.2   Accessibility and Transportation

Although neither Midland-Penetanguishene or London are remote communities and both are well-served by grocery and other food outlets, parents from both communities described difficulty with physically accessing healthy food for their households and how this negatively affected their food choices and children's diets. Problems with accessibility were often related to income. Several participants described their reliance on public transportation for grocery shopping, and noted that some grocery stores were located in areas that were difficult to access via public transit. Some Midland Métis parents mentioned that accessibility was a particular problem for families living in some parts of the area that were poorly served by public transport in general. One First Nations caregiver mentioned that inconvenient access to grocery stores impacted the frequency of her shopping trips:

> Yeah, that's what we do because we don't have a car so we go, like my mom will drive me to the grocery store once a month and then if it [food] goes bad, it goes bad and we just have to wait until next month.

Less frequent grocery shopping also affected food-purchasing behaviour. Oftentimes non-perishable food items were a more economical choice since these foods lasted longer than fresher options. Caregivers acknowledged that non-perishable items tended to be the least nutritious. A First Nations caregiver stated:

> I think it's because sometimes when you buy fruits and vegetables, they tend to, like the shelf-life is not as long as the other foods. We just recently moved to the reserve [adjacent to the city] and you need a vehicle to get to town and buy those foods like every so often [...], and a lot of people that live on the reserve, they go grocery shopping maybe once or twice a month, so they're not able to continuously get fruits and vegetables.

10.3.3   Access to Traditional Foods

In general, caregivers felt that a shift away from more traditional First Nations or Métis diets to a "Western" diet was an important contributing factor to overweight and obesity among their children. Traditional Aboriginal diets were considered nutrient rich compared to children's current diets, which were described using various terms (i.e., "packaged foods", "high carbohydrate", "junk food"), as energy-dense and nutrient-poor.

There were several aspects to the lack of traditional foods in contemporary diets. Several mentioned children's preferences for Western food over wild game, for example. Some caregivers believed that this was because children were not given enough opportunity to develop a preference for traditional foods due to the challenges with accessing and affording these options.

When asked about the availability of traditional food items in their communities, caregivers said that these foods were too expensive or simply unavailable, hence introducing Aboriginal foods at home was a challenge. Although Midland-Penetanguishine is located near what would have been traditional harvesting regions, one Métis caregiver said:

> You can get it, but it's expensive. And not all of the traditional foods are easy to get, like wild game, is not easy to get.

Caregivers felt that one reason for the lack of traditional food in contemporary diets was because of the decline in hunting, trapping, fishing, or gathering activities among the community members themselves. Another reason was the change in communal food practices. Some First Nations caregivers mentioned that the traditional practices regarding sharing food among community members had declined and were not practiced in the city. Others mentioned that knowledge of traditional foods and preparation was endangered, and that young parents, in particular, might not be able to prepare traditional meals for their children, even if the foods were available.

Although they were not common, there were some concerns expressed about the quality of some wild game that could be obtained. In London, one parent indicated that she would not consume the fish caught in the local river because of the fears that it had been contaminated by pollution.

Some community members also pointed out that foods thought of as "traditional" were problematic. "Fry bread" (a deep-fried dough) and "Indian Tacos" (tacos made with fry bread) were mentioned by some First Nations participants as foods that had become associated with First Nations community gatherings, but were neither "traditional" in the sense of being part of First Nations diets before European contact, nor healthy.

10.3.4   Coping Strategies for Food Insecurity

In order to deal with food insecurity and not having enough money for healthy food, caregivers spoke about several different coping strategies. Some caregivers mentioned borrowing money or sharing food as options, however the more commonly identified strategies involved relying on family and community programming.

Parents and caregivers mentioned many different food programs offered in London and Midland-Penetanguishene, including food box programs, food

banks, soup kitchens, school breakfast or lunch programs, church meal programs, community kitchens, community gardens, prenatal nutrition programs,
as well as programs on reserve that were used by some off-reserve First Nations
residents of London. Caregivers reported resorting to these programs if there
was not enough money for food or food at home, and sometimes for obtaining
healthy food options. One participant described a program at his community
church:

> I used to call my church in my old neighbourhood, because I just moved recently,
> and I would go there and they would help me out with a grocery card. You're
> allowed to go there every 3 months, but I would go there about maybe once or
> twice a year when I needed to.

However, participants identified numerous barriers to programming that
either hindered their participation or the programs' effectiveness. Caregivers
specifically spoke about the food box programs and food banks within their
communities. They felt that these programs often had food of poor quality that
was either near to or past its expiration date. In addition to subpar food options,
many caregivers from Midland-Penetanguishene recalled feelings of shame
associated with using food banks:

> It takes a lot to swallow your pride to access these resources, and if you're gonna
> go there and be judged by the person that's there that's supposed to be helping
> you, you know, it's gonna be harder to swallow your pride next time. And we
> are a small community we know people, and you walk through a door and your
> neighbours are sitting there at the table volunteering.

The feelings of judgment exacerbated the stigma caregivers already felt were
associated with receiving food charity. A caregiver from London reflected that
stigma in her comments:

> I think a lot of people take advantage of that, too, the free stuff, the free food and
> everything. The way I see it is a lot of the drug users and alcoholics, they can just
> use their cheque and blow it because they're going to get free stuff. That's the way
> I see it because it seems like there's like, I don't know a lot of people think that, or
> talk about it in a way that it's just the people that use drugs or alcoholics that go
> to these free things all the time, but it's not. But then when people talk about it,
> that's the way they talk about things.

Some parents also noted that the types of fresh foods sometimes provided by food banks or "good food boxes" might require cooking or preparation skills that community members might not have. Describing a woman given a bag of potatoes, a First Nations woman commented:

> She didn't know what to do with it. And some people wouldn't know how to cook [them] so it's that sort of mindset as well that you're not used to having these sorts of foods that you don't know what to do with them.

When asked how community programming could be made more effective, caregivers described several strategies including shifting the focus from the child to a more family-oriented approach:

> I think a lot of focus is put into child health here and there whatever, but if more focus was put on […] the family, promoting more family unit type activities where all took part, whatever their abilities are. I think that would make good, positive change.

Additionally, caregivers felt that programs with an Aboriginal cultural component would encourage overall health for children and their communities:

> I think we need more, um, […] Aboriginal days for example, that when you go there everybody in the community is welcome, not only Métis people. We might not feel comfortable going to something that is mainstream, but mainstream people may not necessarily […] it's that education part again. If we have more community/family things that we have multiple opportunities to try different foods that are healthy and engage with different people.

Overall, caregivers identified numerous barriers faced by families to provide healthy foods for their children. Some of these barriers were exacerbated by underlying problems such as low income within the household, which strongly impacted accessibility and food purchasing options.

10.4   DISCUSSION

This qualitative study helps us to understand the connections between food insecurity and children's diets, and uncovers the importance of income, food security, and coping strategies for the weight status of Aboriginal children. Community members' perspectives elucidate the lived experience of Aboriginal families in urban settings, and how the issue of food insecurity continues to be prevalent even among children living alongside sizable non-Aboriginal populations.

The focus group discussions describe a clear relationship between low income and food insecurity, which participants believed had an adverse impact on their children's diets. Current diet practices were perceived to be an important contributor to high obesity rates among First Nations and Métis children. While caregivers did not use the language, "food insecurity," conversations about not having enough food or money for food, and strategies for coping with these conditions, suggest that food insecurity was present and manifests itself in different ways.

Caregivers discussed poor variety of foods, compromised fruit and vegetable intake, as well as the shift away from traditional foods as examples of how food consumption and purchasing patterns changed with food security status. Food insecurity had a negative impact on children's diets, and many caregivers attributed the rise in overweight and obesity to poor diet quality. The wide range of barriers and facilitators to healthy eating and community programming illustrate some potential opportunities for intervention.

It was somewhat unexpected that accessibility of grocery stores would be a major barrier to healthy eating in the communities studied. Accessibility is often discussed in the literature as a barrier for families living in geographically remote settings or on reserve [35, 36]. In both Midland-Penetanguishene and London, caregivers spoke about difficulties accessing public transit, as well as grocery stores being inconveniently located. However it is important to note that convenience and location were not the main hindrances to healthy food access, rather it was low income that made accessing grocery stores so inconvenient. Many caregivers relied on public transit because they could not afford a car, hence the length or distance of grocery stores trips were affected as a result. Despite living in urban settings where the risk of food insecurity should be relatively lower than geographically remote areas, caregivers' experiences clearly demonstrated that food insecurity persists in these households.

The focus groups confirmed that, at least in the views of the participants, low income and resulting food insecurity are likely to be implicated in the higher risk of obesity among Aboriginal children. The community programs that were mentioned as coping strategies by participants tended to address immediate individual needs, rather than the systematic or structural factors leading to low income, and did not appear to be effective in meeting those needs. While community nutrition programs played an important role in facilitating the accessibility and affordability of healthy foods, caregivers described numerous barriers that affected the effectiveness and outreach of those programs. Although food banks helped ensure an adequate quantity of food within households, the quality was seen as often poor and not culturally appropriate; hence they did not seem to contribute to the healthfulness of families' diets. It was also important to learn that caregivers were not comfortable visiting food banks because of the stigma associated with food charity. This deterred caregivers even in times of need because they felt that they were being discriminated by the volunteers and also ashamed for needing to use the food bank. Although many people report shame associated with using food banks, this stigma is perhaps worse for Aboriginal peoples [37].

Successfully and permanently reducing the health inequities experienced by Aboriginal peoples likely requires a change in the macro-level structural factors that are the fundamental causes of those inequities. In Canada, as elsewhere, these are most likely to be addressed by Aboriginal peoples' political action. However, we also think that local public health programming may play a role in reducing insecurity and therefore the risk of obesity among children. Despite the demonstrated higher risk, there have been relatively few programs or interventions aimed at reducing obesity specifically among Aboriginal children, and most have been conducted in discrete Aboriginal communities rather than in urban areas [38].

Many of these existing programs have targeted changing children's physical activity and eating behaviours. However, the group interviews suggested that effective programming might focus more on addressing the applied skills that are necessary for eating healthy, such as meal preparation and preservation, harvesting, food storage and cooking. Many of these skills may have been lost through residential schooling or lack of access to traditional activities. Programming with a strong cultural component might have more meaningful impact, and caregivers suggested taking a more family-targeted approach rather than placing sole emphasis on children. Importantly, caregivers discussed the importance of healthy living overall because they believed it had the potential to address a wide range of health problems for children in the community. Successful community interventions therefore might take a more holistic approach to health, rather than focusing on a single problem such as obesity.

10.4.1 Study Limitations

Child obesity and food insecurity are both sensitive topics that had to be carefully approached during the focus group discussions. The discussions did not probe too deeply into families' coping strategies and personal experiences of food insecurity to avoid making participants feel uncomfortable. However the facilitator and interview guide questions were still able to obtain important and relevant information on the topic. While one-on-one interviews could have been better for accessing more personal information, focus groups were still a better fit given that the objective was not to gain an understanding of the individual experiences, instead the point was to get a broader understanding of what families and children experienced within those communities. Focus groups allowed caregivers to comment beyond their personal experience and share what they had observed in the community. Additionally, the use of an Indigenous facilitator increased participants' comfort with sharing their views, and many drew from personal experience.

Since the focus groups took place in only two Aboriginal communities in Ontario, results are not generalizable. Although it is important to note that the results are not intended to be generalizable to all Métis and First Nations, or to Aboriginal peoples in general. Instead, they provide some insight into the experience of food insecurity and implications of low-income in urban settings for child health.

10.5   CONCLUSION

Few studies have explored the effects of food insecurity on obesity, and none have focused on Aboriginal children living in urban settings despite the fact that they are among the most severely impacted by these two health concerns. There have also been limited studies exploring this topic using qualitative research methods. The focus group discussions around barriers and facilitators to healthy eating, as well as how these barriers relate to obesity, allowed for the identification of some of the challenges that face Aboriginal families living in urban areas.

The results indicate that these challenges may include issues such as a lack of transportation and access to healthy food, which are related to the underlying problem of low income, but are also exacerbated by local conditions such as a lack of public transportation. A lack of access to traditional foods may be a particular problem for people in urban communities. The results support the idea that interventions to reduce the risk of obesity among urban Aboriginal children may benefit from a focus on improving families' food security, and that those efforts should also consider the unique contexts in which those families live.

Future research should focus on exploring food insecurity and diet quality to better understand the relationship with obesity rates among Aboriginal children. Additional focus group discussions are important to identifying strategies to improve program design and delivery. Larger focus groups would also enable a comparison between Aboriginal communities living in different geographic settings. Overall, caregivers and community members provide valuable insights and expertise regarding barriers and facilitators to their children's health and should be included in conversations regarding Aboriginal-focused program planning and policy.

FOOTNOTES

1. "Reserves" are Crown lands set aside for the use of First Nations. Métis and Inuit peoples have not historically been part of the reserve system.
2. In 2011, 75 % of Status First Nations, 42 % of non-Status First Nations, 71 % of Métis, and 43 % of Inuit lived in urban areas [5]
3. This research was funded by the Canadian Institutes for Health Research, Institute for Aboriginal Peoples' Health Operating Grant RN125827–251526

REFERENCES

1. World Health Organization (WHO). Obesity. WHO 2013, [http://www.who.int/topics/obesity/en/]
2. Roberts KC, Shields M, de Groh M, Aziz A, & Gilbert J. Overweight and obesity in children and adolescents: Results from the 2009 to 2011 Canadian Health Measures Survey (Catalogue no. 82-003-XPE). Statistics Canada. 2012. [http://www.statcan.gc.ca/pub/82-003-x/2012003/article/11706-eng.pdf]
3. Shields, M. Measured obesity: Overweight Canadian children and adolescents. (Catalogue no. 82-620-MWE2005001). Statistics Canada. 2005, [http://www5.statcan.gc.ca/access_acces/archive.action?loc=/pub/82-620-m/2005001/pdf/4193660-eng.pdf]
4. Public Health Agency of Canada (PHAC): Obesity in Canada: A joint report from the Public Health Agency of Canada and the Canadian Institute for Health Information. (Catalogue no. HP5-107/2011E-PDF). PHAC. 2011, [http://www.phac-aspc.gc.ca/hp-ps/hl-mvs/oic-oac/index-eng.php]
5. Aboriginal Affairs and Northern Development Canada (AANDC). Aboriginal Demographics from the 2011 National Household Survey. AANDC. 2013, [https://www.aadnc-aandc.gc.ca/eng/1370438978311/1370439050610]
6. Cooke M, Mitrou F, Lawrence D, Guimond E, Beavon D. Indigenous well-being in four countries: an application of the UNDP's Human Development Index to Indigenous Peoples in Australia, Canada, New Zealand and the United States. BMC Health Hum Rights. 2007;7:9.
7. Gracey M, King M. Indigenous health part 1: determinants and disease patterns. Lancet. 2009;374:65–75.

8. King M, Smith A, Gracey M. Indigenous health part 2: the underlying causes of health. Lancet. 2009;374:76–85.

9. Adams C, Dahl G, Peach I, editors. Métis in Canada: History, identity, law and politics. Edmonton: University of Alberta Press; 2013.

10. Bonesteel, J. Canada's Relationship with Inuit: a history of policy and program development. Statistics Canada. 2006, [http://www.aadnc-aandc.gc.ca/eng/1100100016900/1100100016908]

11. Mitrou F, Cooke M, Lawrence D, Povah D, Mobilia E, Guimond E, et al. Gaps in indigenous disadvantage not closing: a census cohort study of social determinants of health in Australia, Canada, and New Zealand from 1981–2006. BMC Public Health. 2014;14:201.

12. Pendakur K, Pendakur R. Aboriginal income disparity in Canada. Toronto: University of Toronto Press; 2011.

13. Evans W, Wolfe B, Adler N. The SES and health gradient: a brief review of the literature. New York: Russell Sage; 2012.

14. Willows ND, Hanley AJ, Delformier T. A socioecological framework to understand weight-related issues in Aboriginal children in Canada. Appl Physiol Nutr Metab. 2012;37:1–13.

15. Anderson SA. Core Indicators of Nutritional State for Difficult-to-Sample Populations. J Nutr. 1990;120:1559–600.

16. Willows ND, Veugelers P, Raine K, Kuhle S. Prevalence and sociodemographic riskfactors related to household food security in Aboriginal peoples in Canada. Public Health Nutr. 2009;12:1150–6.

17. Health Canada. Household Food Insecurity In Canada in 2007–2008: Key Statistics and Graphics. Health Canada. 2012, [http://hc-sc.gc.ca/fn-an/surveill/nutrition/commun/insecurit/key-stats-cles-2007-2008-eng.php#fnb1]

18. Haman F, Fontaine-Bisson B, Batal M, Imbeault P, Blais JM, Robidoux MA. Obesity and Type 2 Diabetes in Northern Canada's Remote First Nations Communities: The Dietary Dilemma. Int J Obes. 2010;34:24–31.

19. Chan HM, Fediuk K, Hamilton S, Rostas L, Caughey A, Kuhnlein H, et al. Food security in Nunavut, Canada: barriers and recommendations. Int J Circumpol Health. 2006;65:416–31.

20. Health Canada. Canadian Community Health Survey, Cycle 2.2, Nutrition (2004): Income-related household food security in Canada. Health Canada. 2007, [http://www.hc-sc.gc.ca/fn-an/surveill/nutrition/commun/income_food_sec-sec_alim-eng.php#fg33]

21. Cooke MJ, Wilk P, Paul KW, & Gonneville SLH. Predictors of obesity among Métis children: Socio-economic, behavioural, and cultural factors. CJPH. 2013, 104. [http://journal.cpha.ca/index.php/cjph/article/view/3765/2833]

22. Oliver LN, & Hayes MV. Effects of neighbourhood income on reported body mass index: an eight year longitudinal study of Canadian children. BMC Public Health. 2008, [http://www.biomedcentral.com/1471-2458/8/16]

23. Power, EM. Determinants of healthy eating among low-income Canadians. CJPH. 2005, 96. [http://journal.cpha.ca/index.php/cjph/article/view/1504/1693]

24. Kirkpatrick S, Tarasuk V. The relationship between low income and household food expenditure patterns in Canada. Public Health Nutr. 2003;6:589–97.

25. McIntyre L, Glanville T, Raine KD, Dayle JB, Anderson B, Battaglia N. Do low-income lone mothers compromise their nutrition to feed their children? CMAJ. 2003;168:686–91.

26. Kirkpatrick SI, & Tarasuk V. Food insecurity and participation in community food programs among low-income Toronto families. CJPH. 2009, 100. [http://journal.cpha.ca/index.php/cjph/article/view/1771/1955]

27. Power EM. Conceptualizing food security for Aboriginal people in Canada. CJPH. 2008;99:95–7.

28. Statistics Canada. NHS Focus on Geography Series–London. Statistics Canada. 2014, [http://www12.statcan.gc.ca/nhs-enm/2011/as-sa/fogs-spg/Pages/FOG.cfm?lang=E&level=3&GeoCode=555]

29. Statistics Canada. NHS Focus on Geography Series– Midland. http://www12.statcan.gc.ca/nhs-enm/2011/as-sa/fogs-spg/Pages/FOG.cfm?lang=E&level=3&GeoCode=571.

30. Statistics Canada. NHS Focus on Geography Series– Penetanguishene. http://www12.statcan.gc.ca/nhs-enm/2011/as-sa/fogs-spg/Pages/FOG.cfm?lang=E&level=4&GeoCode=3543072.

31. O'Donnell V, & Wallace S. First Nations, Métis and Inuit Women. Statistics Canada. 2011, [http://www.statcan.gc.ca/pub/89-503-x/2010001/article/11442-eng.htm#a15]

32. Statistics Canada. 2011 National Household Survey: Aboriginal Peoples in Canada. Statistics Canada. 2011, [http://www.statcan.gc.ca/daily-quotidien/130508/dq130508a-eng.pdf]

33. NVivo qualitative data analysis software. QSR International Pty Ltd. Version 10. 2013.

34. Miles MB, Huberman AM. Qualitative data analysis: An expanded sourcebook. 2nd ed. Beverley Hills: Sage Publications, Inc; 1994.

35. Elliot B, Jayatilaka D, Brown C, Varley L, & Corbett KK. "We are not being heard": Aboriginal perspectives on traditional foods access and food security. J Environ Public Health. 2012. [http://www.hindawi.com/journals/jeph/2012/130945/]

36. Willows ND. Determinants of healthy eating in Aboriginal peoples in Canada: the current state of knowledge and research gaps. Can J Public Health. 2005;96:S32–41.

37. Hamelin A, Beaudry M, Habicht J. Characterization of household food insecurity in Quebec: food and feelings. Soc Sci Med. 2002;54:119–32.

38. Towns C, Cooke M, Rysdale L, Wilk P. Healthy weights interventions in Aboriginal children and youth: a review of the literature. Can J Diet Pract Res. 2014;75:125–31.

PART V
Conclusion

CHAPTER 11

Household Hardships, Public Programs, and Their Associations with the Health and Development of Very Young Children: Insights from Children's Health Watch

Katherine M. Joyce, Amanda Breen,
Stephanie Ettinger De Cuba, John T. Cook,
Kathleen W. Barrett, Grace Paik, Natasha Rishi,
Bianca Pullen, Ashley Schiffmiller, and
Deborah A. Frank

11.1 EVALUATING FOOD INSECURITY AND HOUSEHOLD HARDSHIPS

Food insecurity, a household-level economic and social condition of limited or uncertain access to adequate food for all household members to live an active and healthy life, is a serious public health problem in the US. This problem waxes and wanes with fluctuations in public policies and economic climate. While the prevalence of household food insecurity has remained fairly stable over the past 2 years, the increase in 2008, the first full year of the recession, was the largest since the national food security survey began in 1995[1] and has not returned to pre-2008 levels.

The most recent US Department of Agriculture (USDA) assessment of food security in the US reported that overall food insecurity numbers (measured by the 18-item US Food Security Scale [FSS][2]) were relatively unchanged from 2009 to 2010, with 14.5% of households (17.2 million) considered food inse-cure; most of those who were food insecure lived inside metropolitan areas.[3] That same year, 21.6% of all US children (16.2 million) lived in food-insecure households. Pediatric clinicians have observed that not only food insecurity but also other material hardships, such as energy and housing insecurity (respec-tively, inadequate home energy availability due to economic constraints and overcrowded living situations or frequent moves), exert a cumulative negative effect on child health.[4]

Many research and advocacy groups use econometrics and/or biostatistics to explore the health and educational effects of food insecurity.[5,6] Children's HealthWatch (formerly known as the Children's Sentinel Nutrition Assessment Program or C-SNAP) is one such group. Children's HealthWatch was founded in 1998 to bring evidence and analysis from the front lines of pediatric care to policy makers and the public. The goal of Children's HealthWatch was to develop a continuous dataset that could monitor child health in real time as eco-nomic conditions and government assistance programs changed. At the time, other researchers collected young children's anthropometric data primarily from datasets of children already receiving benefits from the Special Supplemental Nutrition Program for Women, Infants, and Children (WIC) or Headstart and reflected conditions from 1 to several years before publication.[7]

Some national data collection efforts obtained health information but not data on family hardship or safety-net program participation, while still oth-ers that collected program participation data lacked information on children's health, growth, and development. At present, several important longitudinal studies include the FSS but mostly focus on older children. To our knowl-edge, the Children's HealthWatch dataset is the oldest and largest of children ages 0 to 4 year olds that includes other material hardships, such as energy insecurity.[8-11]

From its inception, the study has focused on a sentinel population[i] of very young children. The rationale for this focus is both scientific and sociological. From a scientific perspective, during the developmental window from birth to preschool, the rapidly increasing size and function of the developing brain demands consistently high levels of nutritional substrate. Deficits in the growth of brain and body following nutritional deprivation or other hardships during this sensitive period, when the foundations of future health and cognitive development are largely determined, are difficult to remediate later in life. Paradoxically, this sensitive period is also the developmental epoch during which children in the US are most likely to live in poverty[12] and least likely to participate in formal child care or educational settings.[13] Thus, children of this age are typically "visible" only to their family members and health care providers.

As a result, the needs of very young children are often not addressed in important policy debates. Consistent with the medical model, Children's HealthWatch focuses on two broad phenomena: 1) the association of one or more exposures (material hardships) to each other and to health outcomes; and 2) the effect of population-level interventions (such as food assistance programs) on reducing the severity or prevalence of the exposure or reducing the negative health impact of the exposure. Monitoring and reporting on the association of these factors with the well-being of the youngest children lends this constituency a voice in matters of policy that will eventually impact their potential to be healthy and productive adults.

Children's HealthWatch monitors the impact of food insecurity alone and in conjunction with other hardships common to low-income families; these hardships include energy insecurity, housing insecurity, and constrained access to health care. Such research evaluates systematically the common-sense notion that ready access to sufficient healthful food, safe and stable housing, and adequate household energy resources can position young children on a trajectory for health and success in school and, later, in the workforce.

This paper explores Children's HealthWatch's research methods, selected findings, and examples of diverse approaches to dissemination of these findings in professional settings, national and local reports and briefs, and legislative testimony. An exhaustive list of this work can be found at www.childrenshealthwatch.org.

11.2   CHILDREN'S HEALTHWATCH—ANALYTIC FOCUS

Though the 18 items that comprise the FSS are essentially unchanged, the category in which an individual fits according to how he or she scores on the scale has varied over time; these variations have resulted in several possible classifications describing a household's or individual's experience with access to food.[14] The FSS also includes 8 child-focused items to measure food security specifically among children.[15] The terms "food insecure" and "food secure" are the broad categories used to describe experience with food as determined by the FSS and are described in Table 1.

TABLE 11.1   Changes in Description of Food Security[16]

USDA Pre-2006 Label	USDA Current Label	Description of Conditions in the Household, per Food Security Survey
Food security	High food security	No reported indications of food- access problems or limitations
	Marginal food security	One or two reported indications— typically of anxiety over food sufficiency or shortage of food in the house; little or no indication of changes in diets or food intake
Food insecurity without hunger	Low food security	Reports of reduced quality, variety, or desirability of diet; little or no indication of reduced food intake
Food insecurity with hunger	Very low food security	Reports of multiple indications of disrupted eating patterns and reduced food intake

Most frontline providers continue to use the common-sense pre- 2006 terms rather than low and very low food security. Children's HealthWatch analyses use the conservative approach of 3 endorsed items on the FSS to refer to a family as "food insecure" while some groups interpret food insecurity at the marginal food secure level or use alternate scoring systems.[17] Children's HealthWatch uses the scoring system of the USDA's Economic Research Service (ERS) to divide households into 3 mutually exclusive categories: 1) food secure on the 18-item FSS; 2) food insecure on the household scale but food secure on the child scale; and 3) food insecure on the household scale and the child scale. (See Table 2)

TABLE 11.2   Levels of Food Security and Insecurity[18]

Level of Food Insecurity	Assessing Status Using the FSS
Food secure on the household and child scale	Household reports 0 to 2 indications of food insecurity to the entire set of 18 questions
Food insecure on the household scale but food secure on the child scale	Household reports 3 or more indications of food insecurity in response to the entire set of 18-questions
Food insecure on the household scale and the child scale	Household reports 2 or more of the child-referenced questions (11-18) of the FSS

11.3   CHILDREN'S HEALTHWATCH STUDY SAMPLE COMPOSITION

Children's HealthWatch currently collects data through one-on-one surveys between trained interviewers and caregivers of patients under the age of 4 in emergency departments or primary care clinics in 5 US cities. Since 1998, over 42,000 households have completed the survey at one of the 7 research sites listed below. Each of the sites is located in a predominantly low-income area and has an affiliated multidisciplinary clinic to provide care to underweight young children, including those identified in the course of research procedures. Each site has approval for human subjects research from its Institutional Review Board (IRB), and all studies have been conducted with IRB approval in place.

Data collection sites are:

- University of Maryland School of Medicine, Baltimore, Maryland
- Boston Medical Center, Boston, Massachusetts
- Arkansas Children's Hospital, Little Rock, Arkansas
- Hennepin County Medical Center, Minneapolis, Minnesota
- St. Christopher's Hospital for Children, Philadelphia, Pennsylvania Inactive sites (due to insufficient funding) are:
- Harbor UCLA Medical Center Torrance, Los Angeles, California (inactive as of 2001)
- Mary's Center for Maternal and Child Care, Washington, DC (inactive as of 2000)

Caregivers interviewed by Children's HealthWatch comprise a sentinel cross-sectional convenience sample. Interviewers survey caregiver-child dyads consenting to participation in the survey and meeting the following inclusion criteria: 1) patient is <48 months of age and seeking care at acute or primary care clinics or hospital emergency departments; 2) caregiver lives in the state where the interview is being conducted; 3) the interview can be conducted verbally in English, Spanish, or (Minneapolis only) Somali; 4) the household has not participated in the Children's HealthWatch survey in the previous 6 months; and 5) the caregiver lives with the child and has full knowledge of the child's life. Caregivers of critically ill or injured children are not approached.

In early 2011, the eligible child age range was broadened from 0 to 36 months to 0 to 48 months in an effort to expand the sample to an age group where the risk of obesity increases and developmental findings better predict school readiness.

11.4   THE CHILDREN'S HEALTHWATCH SURVEY

Each caregiver completes one full survey during his or her child's visit to the emergency department or primary care center. While the survey has been modified slightly over time to accommodate changes in policy and research questions, the areas of focus generally include the following:

Data acquired through medical record review and/or anthropometric measurement:

- Child's dehydration and hospital admission status on the day of interview
- Child's current height and weight (at some sites, measurements are taken by clinical staff; at others, the interviewers use standardized protocols to measure children)

Data acquired through caregiver report:

- Developmental assessment (Parents' Evaluation of Development Status[19]) and use of Early Intervention services
- Demographic background
- Caregiver and household employment status, income, and use of child care
- Child's health history, including lifetime hospitalizations and health insurance coverage
- Household access to medical care and healthcare trade-offs
- Caregiver health questions, including the Kemper Depression Screener[20] (female caregivers only), and maternal/paternal anthropometric measurements

- Evaluation of housing security
- Evaluation of energy security
- The USDA FSS[15]
- Participation in public assistance programs including Supplemental Nutrition Assistance Program (SNAP, formerly The Food Stamp Program), WIC, Temporary Assistance for Needy Families (TANF), energy assistance such as Low-Income Home Energy Assistance Program (LIHEAP), and housing subsidies, such as Section 8 and public housing.

At the end of every interview, the caregiver is offered outreach services that differ by site, ranging from a list of community resources and WIC offices to follow-up from an outreach worker. Caregivers are also offered the chance to be contacted for media or legislative testimony opportunities. Small incentives—for example, supermarket gift cards or a toy for the child—are provided.

11.5   SURVEY ANALYSIS

All data from the Children's HealthWatch survey are maintained and analyzed at the Boston University School of Public Health's Data Coordinating Center. Every 6 months, a new batch of clean data is added to the dataset. There is no "typical" data analysis in Children's HealthWatch. Each analysis includes (at a minimum) descriptive statistics, bivariate associational measures, and multivariate analyses adjusted for potential confounding factors. Propensity score matching may also be used. Because the study is ongoing, with some measures being added or omitted over time and sites joining and leaving the project, different publications from different periods described below have varying sample sizes depending on how many participants had been interviewed at the time of the analysis. In addition, some papers focus only on subsamples selected from the overall sample to answer specific questions.

11.6   MONITORING CHILDREN'S HEALTH ON THE FRONT LINES OF CARE

Federal and state programs exist to support households struggling with the costs of basic needs, but there can be logistical and bureaucratic barriers to program participation. Moreover, some discretionary programs lack funding to support all those who are eligible.[ii] Children's HealthWatch examines the health effects of nutrition assistance programs, including SNAP, WIC, and programs that indirectly fight food insecurity, such as energy assistance programs and subsidized housing, described in Table 3. Of these programs, only SNAP is an entitlement program, designed to serve all eligible people who apply. Discretionary programs, on the other hand, are vulnerable to budget cuts year to year. When funding for discretionary programs is cut at the federal level, individual states create criteria to determine which families will receive assistance. Some states use their own budgets to supplement the needs of programs so that every eligible family receives assistance. In other cases, assistance may be provided on a first-come, first-served basis.

TABLE 11.3   Selection of Federal Assistance Programs

Federal Program	Description
Supplemental Nutrition Assistance Program (SNAP)	Formerly called the Food Stamp Program, SNAP is an entitlement program; households are provided a monthly allotment for food purchases on an Electronic Benefits Transfer card.
Temporary Assistance for Needy Families (TANF)	Program that provides monthly cash benefits to very low-income families based on eligibility standards established by the state within federal guidelines. Recipient families must fulfill ongoing work and other requirements, and there is a time limit on benefits.
Special Supplemental Nutrition Program for Women, Infants, and Children (WIC)	Discretionary program that provides nutrient-dense foods to income-eligible pregnant, postpartum, and lactating women and children up to the age of 5.
Low Income Home Energy Assistance Program (LIHEAP)	Energy assistance program that provides funds for heating costs, often on a first-come, first-served basis.
Section 8 and Public Housing	Two of the types of housing subsidies available to individuals at low-income levels; eligible families sometimes spend multiple years on waiting lists before receiving the subsidy.

11.7   OVERVIEW OF FINDINGS

Children's HealthWatch and others have found that, while food insecurity at both the household and child levels has a negative impact on child health outcomes, other hardships also come into play. These hardships, such as food insecurity, may be modified by participation in public assistance programs. All families, but particularly those who have limited incomes and young children, are constantly juggling the costs of paying for basic needs like food, shelter, household utilities, and medical care. A change in one affects the others; parents, despite the best of intentions, have to make difficult decisions whether to pay for a child's prescription, buy nutrient-dense food, or allocate scarce financial resources to rent or utility bills. Supports—including housing subsidies, WIC, and energy assistance—can offset some costs and free resources for other needs, in turn allowing parents to do more to promote their children's food security and health.

11.8 EXAMINATION OF FOOD INSECURITY IN CHILDREN'S HEALTHWATCH POPULATIONS

Children's HealthWatch and others have concluded that household and child food insecurity have negative impacts on child health.[21,22] Analysis by other groups suggests that the threshold for adverse health or developmental effects may actually be lower than previously thought (i.e., even a marginal score on the FSS may correlate with poor outcomes).[23,24] As outlined in more detail in the following sections, Children's HealthWatch analyses have found that food insecurity puts children at a higher risk for iron-deficiency and iron-deficiency anemia, lifetime hospitalizations, fair or poor health, and developmental concerns. It should be noted that Gundersen and Kreider[25] observed that in samples like those of Children's HealthWatch, it is more likely that the negative health impacts of food insecurity have been underreported rather than overreported.

11.9 HISTORY OF HOSPITALIZATIONS AND REPORT OF FAIR/POOR HEALTH RELATED TO FOOD INSECURITY

The survey includes questions about the child's hospitalizations since birth and the caregiver's rating of his or her child's health status.[iii] In a variety of analyses using the Children's HealthWatch dataset, children living in food insecure households are more likely to have been hospitalized and to have their health reported as fair or poor (versus excellent or good) than their counterparts living in food secure households. A 2004 study aimed to determine whether household food insecurity is associated with adverse health outcomes in the Children's HealthWatch sample.[21] In the sample of 11,539 children under 36 months old, interviewed between 1998 and 2002, 21.4% were food insecure. Although household SNAP benefit receipt attenuated associations between food insecurity and the child's fair or poor health status, the odds of fair or poor health in children living in food insecure households remained almost twice that of children in food secure households [AOR=1.90, 95% CI=1.66-2.18][iv] even after controlling for SNAP participation. The odds of hospitalization since birth among the children in food insecure homes were more than 30% higher than those of the children in food secure homes [AOR =1.31 95% CI=1.16-1.48] and not modified by SNAP participation.

In 2006, further analyses addressed child as well as household food insecurity. In a sample of 17,158 child-caregiver dyads, 10% reported only household-level food insecurity, and 12% reported child food insecurity in addition to household-level food insecurity. Adjusted analyses revealed child-level food insecurity increased the adjusted odds of negative child health outcomes compared to household food insecurity with children food secure [AOR 1.51 v AOR 1.99-2.00].[18]

While data specific to the reason for prior hospitalizations are not collected, these findings suggest that an increase in food insecurity is correlated with an increased likelihood of history of hospitalization for young children. The average charge[v] in 2009 of a single hospitalization for a child under 1 for any reason was $13,300. The average charge for a single hospitalization for a child aged 1-4 was $21,045.[26] Hospital fees are paid through a number of streams, including the individual, insurance (i.e., public and private), or at times, the hospital that provided the care. None of these figures, however, include rehabilitation, follow-up care, or home care costs. [27]

11.10   IRON-DEFICIENCY ANEMIA AND FOOD INSECURITY

Iron-deficiency anemia has been correlated with impaired cognitive, mental and psychomotor development and diminished immune response in children.[29,30] Children's HealthWatch wanted to determine if a relationship exists between anemia and food insecurity in the study population. Two independent analyses at Children's HealthWatch sites combined survey results with hematological data collected in retrospective chart reviews to explore iron-deficiency, iron-deficiency anemia, and food insecurity in the study population. Children eligible for both analyses received primary care at the respective medical centers and had appropriate lab values available in their medical records.

Researchers examined the association between child-level food insecurity and iron status among the Boston sample. Though interviews at Boston Medical Center were conducted exclusively in the Emergency Department, many of these patients used Boston Medical Center as their medical home for primary care. As a result, researchers were able to collect retrospectively appropriate lab measures for 626 children over the age of 6 months at the time of their interview between June 1996 and May 2001.

Box 1: Key Findings: Iron-deficiency Anemia and Food Insecurity

- Food insecure young children were at 2.4 times greater risk of having irondeficiency anemia compared to their food secure peers

---

In the final sample (n=626), 7% had iron deficiency without anemia, and 11% had iron-deficiency anemia. Adjusting for confounding variables, food insecure children had 2.4 greater odds of having iron-deficiency anemia [AOR, 2.4; 95% CI, 1.1-5.2, p=0.02] compared to food secure children.31 In other words, food insecure children were at 2.4 times greater risk for irreversible pathophysiologic effects of iron deficiency that might leave them more developmentally at-risk than their food secure peers—all by 3 years of age. The threshold for this effect was child food insecurity, not household food insecurity alone, suggesting a dose response of nutritional deprivation.

The second study examined a sample of 2,853 children in Minneapolis and focused on the relationship between anemia and household (as opposed to child) food security. In this study, levels of food insecurity were divided into 3 renamed categories (as explained above): high/marginal food security, low food security, and very low food security (which encompasses child food insecurity). Children younger than 36 months old living in households with very low food security were almost twice as likely to have iron-deficiency anemia compared with those in food secure households, independent of age, gender, WIC participation, race/ethnicity, US-born status, breast feeding, health insurance type, and plasma lead concentration [AOR=1.98, 95% CI 1.11, 3.53].[32]

11.11 CHILD DEVELOPMENT AND FOOD INSECURITY

Children's HealthWatch research found that young children from food insecure households are more likely to be at developmental risk in early childhood. Such risk is an early warning sign for lack of readiness for school. The Parents' Evaluation of Developmental Status (PEDS)[19] used to evaluate children from birth to 8 years of age was introduced to the survey in 2004 and is administered to all caregivers with children who are at least 4 months old, the age at which the screen becomes more readily interpretable. In addition, caregivers are asked about their children's current or past enrollment in Early Intervention programs, regardless of age. To assist detection of developmental disabilities, the PEDS consists of 10 questions that assess cognition, expressive and receptive language, fine and gross motor behavior, socioemotional development, self-help, and learning.[33] Even after excluding families reporting food insecurity with hunger and controlling for multiple potential confounders, analysis showed children in food insecure families were significantly more likely than those in food secure households to screen positive on the PEDS [AOR 1.77, 95% CI 1.23-2.56].[34] The effects of food insecurity on early childhood development may be explained through both nutritive and non-nutritive pathways. Families experiencing food insecurity and constrained by finances often choose less expensive, calorie-dense but nutrient-poor foods to maximize satiety for all household members. This compromise can result in a deficiency of micronutrients (as suggested by the association of food insecurity and anemia described above), a deficiency which may alter children's developing neurotransmitters.[35]

Maternal depression is prevalent in our data set and is among the impor-tant non-nutritive pathways by which food insecurity impacts child develop-ment. Among 5,306 mothers in Children's HealthWatch data who completed the maternal depression screen from 2000 to 2001, 35% had positive reports of depressive symptoms.[36] Mothers with depressive symptoms were more likely to report household food insecurity [AOR: 2.69; 95% CI: 2.33–3.11] than moth-ers without depressive symptoms. Mothers with depressive symptoms were also more likely to have had their TANF benefits reduced [AOR: 1.52; 95% CI: 1.03–2.25] and to have lost SNAP benefits [AOR: 1.56; 95% CI: 1.06 –2.30] but not WIC than mothers who did not report depressive symptoms. Lastly, mothers with depressive symptoms were more likely to report that their chil-dren were at developmental risk on the PEDS, but the association of food inse-curity with the child's developmental risk was robust after controlling for the mother's depressive symptoms.[34] Other literature reports strong links between maternal depression and adverse child development outcomes. For example, both maternal depression and paternal depression have been shown to have negative impacts on child development.[37] However, whether family hardships such as food insecurity caused depressive symptoms or depressive symptoms caused hardships cannot be answered by cross-sectional datasets like Children's HealthWatch.

11.12   SNAP AND WIC DECREASE FOOD INSECURITY AND ATTENUATE ITS IMPACT ON CHILDREN'S OUTCOMES

Multiple research groups conclude that governmental assistance programs reduce food insecurity and support children's health.[38-40] Using data from the longitudinal Three-City Study where at least one child had to be 0 to 4 years old or 10 to 14 years old, DePolt et al41 concluded that participation in SNAP is likely associated with fewer food hardships. Though governmental assistance programs do not entirely eliminate food insecurity, they may attenuate the negative impacts. Knowing that food insecurity leads to fair/poor health outcomes, Children's HealthWatch researchers investigated whether or not SNAP receipt—a logical remedy for food insecurity—modified effects of food insecurity among a sample of 11,539 caregivers, 21.4% of whom reported household food insecurity.[21] A dose-response relation appeared between fair/poor health status and severity of food insecurity. Looking at food insecurity as a dichotomous predictor (food-secure v food-insecure), children living in food-insecure households had nearly twice as great odds of having their health status reported as "fair/poor" as those for similar children in food-secure households [AOR1.90, 95% CI: 1.66–2.18]. When the sample was analyzed by severity of food insecurity, children in households categorized as food insecure without hunger had odds of health being reported fair/poor greater than those in food-secure households [AOR 1.73, 95% CI: 1.48-2.02] and children in households that were food insecure with hunger were even more likely to be reported as being in fair/poor health compared to children in food-secure households [AOR 2.31, 95% CI 1.89- 2.82]. Sub-analysis showed that being in food insecure household increased the odds of fair/poor health by 2.11 times among children in households eligible for but not receiving SNAP benefit In comparison, those children living in food insecure families who received SNAP benefits had increased odds of fair/poor health 1.52 times greater than those in food secure families—a much lower level of risk.[21] In the Children's HealthWatch sample, receipt of SNAP has an especially powerful positive effect for children of immigrants—a group whose level of poverty and food insecurity is consistently higher than the general population. Children of immigrant parents who receive SNAP benefits are 32% less likely to be in poor health than children of immigrant parents whose families do not receive them.[42]

11.13 BARRIERS TO ACCESSING ASSISTANCE PROGRAMS ASSOCIATED WITH POOR HOUSEHOLD AND CHILD OUTCOMES

Although SNAP is an entitlement program, there are families who may be eligible for SNAP but do not receive the benefit due to access barriers. Barriers to SNAP participation reported by Children's HealthWatch families included not having information about the program, being too young to be head of household for SNAP benefits, having concerns about the bureaucratic hassle of applying for SNAP, administrative issues like missing deadlines, and immigration concerns. Those families who were eligible for but did not receive SNAP because of one or more of these access barriers were found to have a greater likelihood of experiencing food insecurity at the household and child levels, experiencing housing insecurity, and needing to make trade-offs between medical care and basic needs like paying for rent, utilities, or food.[43] Children were not the only ones who felt the ill effects of barriers to the program. Female caregivers in families who experienced access barriers to SNAP were more likely to report having depressive symptoms.

Even when a family receives SNAP, the maximum level of benefits is rarely enough to purchase sufficient healthful food each month. The maximum SNAP benefit is calculated on the basis of the cost of the Thrifty Food Plan, established by USDA scientists as a nutritionally adequate diet at the lowest possible cost.[44] The 2008 report, *Coming Up Short: High Food Costs Outstrip Food Stamp Benefits*[45] (based on a pilot study in Boston[46]), examined the accessibility and affordability of food items on the Thrifty Food Plan shopping list and more healthy food items in corner stores, medium-sized stores, and supermarkets in Boston and Philadelphia. In November 2011, the study was updated with data from Philadelphia in a report entitled *The Real Cost of a Healthy Diet: 2011.*[47] In all versions of this study and at both sites, we found that the maximum SNAP allotment for a family of 4 was not sufficient to purchase the items on the Thrifty Food Planvi market basket shopping list in any size store.

Unlike SNAP, WIC is not an entitlement program. WIC serves 53% of all babies born in the US. Despite the program's wide reach among infants and health and development benefits for young children, nationally only 57% of all eligible children and women received WIC from 1994 to 2003.[48] A number of studies[49-51] have demonstrated the positive effect of WIC participation during pregnancy on infant outcomes. Less is known about postnatal participation. Children's HealthWatch found that receipt of WIC for children under 3 is associated with a greater likelihood of the children being in good health, being food secure, and having a healthy weight and height for their age compared to peers who were eligible for but did not receive WIC due to access barriers. In addition, receipt of WIC was associated with decreased risk of developmental delay among children under the age of 3 when compared to children whose mothers reported access barriers to WIC. Mothers in the Children's HealthWatch sample reported that the most common barriers were limited WIC office hours, problems with transportation, difficulty getting to the WIC office to pick up vouchers, and the lack of a permanent address.[52]

11.14 HOUSING INSECURITY: CHILD HEALTH OUTCOMES AND HOUSING SUBSIDY PROGRAMS

The work of Children's HealthWatch is often guided by the experience of our clinicians. Our pediatricians heard over and over from patient families in clinic that housing stability was having a direct impact on their young children. Thus, evaluation of "housing security" was introduced into the Children's HealthWatch survey. There is no simple, widely used federal definition of "housing instability" or "housing insecurity." The US Department of Health and Human Services defines "housing insecurity" as "high housing costs in proportion to income, poor housing quality, unstable neighborhoods, overcrowding, or homelessness." Children's HealthWatch, however, operationalizes the concept as 3 conditions short of outright homelessness: crowded, doubled up, and multiple moves in the past year.[53] A relatively small proportion of the Children's HealthWatch sample (approximately 5%) report that they are homeless or do not have a steady place to sleep at night. However, almost half fit the more inclusive term of "housing insecurity." Of an overall sample of non-homeless eligible caregiver-child dyads (n=22,069), 46% experienced "housing insecurity." Within the definition of housing insecurity, we define 2 groups: crowding (more than 2 people per bedroom) or doubling up (living temporarily with other families because of economic difficulties), referred to collectively as "crowding," and multiple moves (2 or more moves in past year). In this cohort, 9% of families with secure housing reported household food insecurity, compared to 12% of overcrowded families and 16% of those with multiple moves. After considering multiple potential confounding characteristics, children living in overcrowded housing were more likely than housing secure children to experience household and child food insecurity; those in households that had multiple moves had increased risks of household and child food insecurity as well as fair/poor child health and developmental delays. While neither household nor child food insecurity alone predicted poor anthropometric outcomes in previous studies, in these analyses multiple moves were associated with lower weight for age z scores [AOR= -0.082 vs. -0.013, p=.02].[53] Children living with both housing and food insecurity face a dual threat to their health and development.

Children's HealthWatch has begun to explore, but not yet published in peer-reviewed journals, an alternate indicator of housing stress not covered by the housing insecurity definition delineated above. Compared to families who have not reported problems paying the rent or mortgage on time in the last year, families who were behind on rent or mortgage more frequently experienced food and/or energy insecurity and made more trade-offs between housing, utilities, food, or other expenses to pay medical bills.

Children's HealthWatch twice evaluated the impact of subsidized housing as a treatment for the adverse health effects associated with housing insecurity. Housing subsidies limit the amount paid by families for rent to 30% of their income with the remainder made up by the subsidy. Subsidized Housing and Children's Nutritional Status, [54] published in June 2005, examined the relationship between food security and child health among children living in subsidized housing compared to children in families renting apartments at market rates, but whose eligibility for subsidized housing was indicated by their acceptance onto a waiting list for such housing. Children living in families on the wait list for subsidized housing had lower weight-for-age scores than children living in subsidized housing. More recently, Rx for Hunger: Affordable Housing[55] focused on solutions to the findings that children living in subsidized housing were more likely to be food secure and less likely to be seriously underweight (<5th percentile weight-for-age according to Centers for Disease Control/National Center for Health Statistics growth criteria) than children whose families were on the wait list for subsidized housing.

11.15   ENERGY INSECURITY: CHILD HEALTH OUTCOMES AND ENERGY ASSISTANCE PROGRAMS

Proper heating or cooling in a child's environment is particularly important to the youngest children whose high surface area to mass ratio creates poor thermoregulation abilities and thus makes them extraordinarily vulnerable to extreme heat and cold. Such young children may not be able to express verbally when they are hot or cold. A Boston study, which was a precursor to Children's HealthWatch, reported a lower weight-for-age in children seeking emergency hospital care within 3 months following the coldest month of the year than all children seeking care the rest of the year.[56] Contributing to these physiological processes is the "heat or eat" dilemma—a quandary well known to families and their physicians in resource-poor areas. Low-income families must often decide between paying to heat their home during the winter or buying food for their family. Even if heat is not the particular issue, other utilities may be—affecting refrigeration for food, electricity to plug in a nebulizer for an asthmatic child, or a phone line to receive calls about job interviews. If a family must choose between keeping a warm house and lights on or eating a nutritious meal, sometimes nutrition suffers.

To measure this phenomenon, the Children's HealthWatch research team empirically developed and published a research indicator for household energy security defined as a household experiencing at least 1 of the following conditions within the previous year: moderate energy insecurity (a threatened utility shut-off or refusal to deliver heating fuel) and severe energy insecurity (an actual utility shut-off or refused delivery of heating fuel, an unheated or uncooled day because of the inability to pay utility bills, or the use of a cooking stove as a source of heat). Findings showed that household energy insecurity strongly correlated with household and child food insecurity, with the relationship intensifying with the severity of the energy insecurity. Those in households with severe energy insecurity had odds of household food insecurity 3 times as great as those in energy secure households [AOR=3.06 95% CI: 2.46–3.81]. Even moderate energy insecurity (threatened but not actually shut-off) was associated with greater odds of household food insecurity, child food insecurity, child fair/poor health, and hospitalization since birth.[57]

Children's HealthWatch also assessed the potential policy "treatment" for energy insecurity—the federal program, LIHEAP—which assists households with home energy expenses. In the 2006 article, "Heat or Eat: The Low Income Home Energy Assistance Program and Nutritional and Health Risks Among Children Less Than 3 Years of Age,"[58] researchers looked at the growth measurements and health of children living in families receiving and not receiving LIHEAP. Covariate adjusted analyses indicated fewer children living in households receiving energy assistance were underweight (p-value=.01) or were admitted from the emergency room visit compared to those living in similar households not receiving energy assistance [AOR=1.32; 95% CI=1.00–1.74]. However, there was no increase in overweight among children in households receiving versus not receiving energy assistance. More recent findings have shown that families who received energy assistance were also 14% more likely to be housing secure than those without assistance from LIHEAP. [59]

11.16   RECEIPT OR LOSS OF BENEFITS AND IMPACT ON FOOD INSECURITY AND CHILDREN'S OUTCOMES

SNAP and WIC are not the only programs that modulate the odds of experiencing food insecurity or the effects of food insecurity. A report prepared by Children's HealthWatch for the Joint Center on Political and Economic Studies in 2006, *The Impact of Food Insecurity on the Development of Young Low-Income Black and Latino Children*[60], indicated that TANF, WIC, subsidized housing, SNAP, and energy assistance mitigated the effect of food insecurity on the health and growth of lowincome black children. Similarly, low-income Latino children whose families received TANF, WIC, subsidized housing, or SNAP were more likely to be food secure than their low-income peers who did not receive these benefits. WIC receipt, in particular, was linked to healthy weightand height-for-age in both black and Latino children.[60] Conversely, for black children, reductions in TANF left children 56% more likely to be food insecure while sanctions made them 78% more likely to be food insecure, when compared to black children in families that had not had benefits reduced or sanctioned. Similar results in benefit reduction or sanctions were seen in SNAP; for black children in families with a reduction in benefits, infants and toddlers were 33% more likely to be food insecure, while those children in families with sanctioned benefits were 84% more likely to be food insecure. For Latino children, the effects were more severe. Latino children whose caregivers experienced sanctions in SNAP or reductions in TANF were twice as likely to be food insecure than Latino children who did not experience such changes to household benefits. Latino children whose family TANF benefit was sanctioned were 63% more likely to be food insecure.

The loss of governmental program benefits, whether due to sanctions or to losing eligibility because of higher incomes, can also be associated with increased levels of child food insecurity and, in turn, poor child health outcomes. Young children whose families lost SNAP or TANF benefits because their incomes increased above the maximum level of income eligibility more frequently experienced food insecurity than those who remained on SNAP or TANF. The phenomenon of being worse off after marginally gaining income but losing benefits is called the "cliff effect." In the September 2010 Policy Action Brief *Earning*

More, Receiving Less: Loss of Benefits and Child Hunger,[61] Children's HealthWatch reported that, within the Children's HealthWatch sample, the rate of child food insecurity among those currently receiving SNAP was 6.9%, while among families that had lost SNAP benefits due to an increase in income, the rate was 8.9%. Similarly, those who lost TANF benefits due to an increase in income had higher rates of child food insecurity than those currently receiving benefits.

Calculating a Family Hardship Score

Step 1: Families are assigned a score of 0, 1 or 2 for each component (food, energy and housing insecurity) depending on how they respond to a set of questions. They receive a score of 0 if they do not experience insecurity for that component, a score of 1 if they experience moderate insecurity for that component and a score of 2 if they experience it at a severe level.

Step 2: Their scores are summed across the three components to arrive at a total hardship score. A family's level of hardship is then characterized by their total score.

A total score of 0   No Hardship
A total score of 1-3   Moderate Hardship
A total score of 4-6   Severe Hardship

Example: A family could be moderately food insecure (score = 1), severely housing insecure (score = 2) and moderately energy insecure (score = 1) for a total score of 4. This score would place them in the Severe Hardship category.

FIGURE 11.1

11.17 CUMULATIVE MATERIAL HARDSHIPS

Growing out of the understanding that material hardships are interrelated, the Cumulative Hardship Index (see graphic) was developed by the Children's HealthWatch research group, along with an analogous composite indicator of child wellness. The 3 included hardships are food, housing, and energy insecurity. The index was developed by examining a subset of our larger sample (7,141 participants at the 5 active study sites between July 2004 and December 2007).[4] The composite indicator of child wellness synthesizes measures of growth, health, and developmental risk. Findings were replicated in a yet unpublished analysis of a Children's Healthwatch Cohort recruited after 2007.

A "well child" was defined by caregiver report and medical record review as:

- Good to excellent heath • No hospitalizations since birth • Not identified as developmentally "at risk" on the PEDS
- Weight-for-age > 5th percentile < 95th percentile
- Weight-for-height > 10th percentile < 95th percentile
- BMI < 85th percentile for children > 24 months of age

Children's HealthWatch concluded, "increasing levels of a composite measure of remediable adverse material conditions correlated with decreasing adjusted odds of wellness among young US children."[4] In other words, children who experience more than 1 of these hardships suffer greater health and developmental risks than children who experience only 1 hardship. After this work was published,[4] findings were presented in the report *Healthy Families in Hard Times: Solutions for Multiple Family Hardships*[62] to make these results accessible to and useful for policy and advocacy audiences.

We turn now from summarizing various print methods of dissemination of Children's HealthWatch findings (peer-reviewed journal articles for other scientists and reports and briefs for advocates, policy makers, and the general public) to an example of how the work can be synthesized with clinical anecdote and used in the setting of policy formation from legislative hearings to assessment of the effects of a policy change.

11.18 EVIDENCE-BASED CONGRESSIONAL TESTIMONY FROM CHILDREN'S HEALTHWATCH, EXAMPLE JULY 2008

The scientific evidence produced by Children's HealthWatch is disseminated in a wide variety of settings, including legislative hearings. In at least one instance, once a policy suggested by this research was adopted, subsequent research efforts permitted rapid evaluation of its effectiveness.

On July 23, 2008,[63] Congressman Joe Baca of California called to order the hearing of the House of Representatives Subcommittee on Department Operations, Oversight, Nutrition, and Forestry to review the short- and long-term costs of hunger in America. He stated:

Good morning to all of you. And thank you for being here with the Subcommittee to examine the short and long term costs of hunger and that is a very important subject now as we look at what is going on in our country. I am especially grateful to our outstanding witnesses for making the effort to be here today. I appreciate your willingness to educate us. And I state to "educate us" on the result of various studies you have conducted. And the more education we receive, the better, more knowledgeable we are in dealing with the problem.[64]

Included on the panel of policy and public health experts was Dr Diana B. Cutts, a pediatrician at Hennepin County Medical Center in Minneapolis, MN, and Co-Principal Investigator for Children's HealthWatch. By representing our work, she spoke on behalf of the thousands of families who participated in this survey and informed Congress—in accessible but scientific terms—about the direct, positive impact of the nutrition assistance programs under legislative consideration on the bodies and brains of babies and toddlers in the US. Other witnesses included representatives from the Food Research and Action Center, the USDA, California Food Policy Advocates, the Harvard University School of Public Health, and the Schneider Institutes for Health Policy at Brandeis University.

Synthesizing Children's HealthWatch findings and her personal experience as a pediatrician, Dr Cutts elucidated the relationship between food insecurity, its harmful health effects, and the protective buffer that nutrition assistance programs can provide. Dr Cutts also described the clinical manifestations of hunger. By describing the increased vulnerability to chronic illness and infection in one particular patient and citing Children's HealthWatch findings on thousands of food insecure households with young children, she illuminated for the committee how science was very real in the lives of her patients. Children's HealthWatch research findings were used to make clear this connection was not only the anecdotal experience of a single pediatrician. She stated:

> Children from food insecure households are 30% more likely to be hospitalized because of their diminished reserve and vulnerability in the face of typical childhood illness....these kids can't just bounce back because their immune systems are so depressed from inadequate nutrition that they often begin a cycle of weight loss and recurrent infections that then perpetuate each other.

Dr Cutts also described the personal stories of several children living in food insecure households, some of whom have conditions illustrated in Children's HealthWatch publications, including anemia and developmental delays.

Dr Cutts described how household hardships compound medical problems as she told the story of the family of a recently hospitalized 5-year-old asthmatic child who could not afford the child's medications because they needed to pay for food, utilities, and rent. After connecting the dots between policy and child health for the committee, Dr Cutts suggested a practical application of Children's HealthWatch's findings through federal policy. She stated:

> Do all of my patients' ills stem from food insecurity? Of course not. But, my reality is that for more than a third of them, food insecurity is a constant companion to their health, directly and indirectly influencing it in both immediate and distant ways. . . . But my reach as their doctor is typically one child, one family at a time. Your reach spans the country and I urge you to think of our time together in clinic and boldly work to create programs and policies that promote healthy and bright futures for all children. For example, I know that Congress is considering another economic stimulus package; I encourage you to make a temporarily increased food stamp benefit part of the package, as it would do so much to directly help the children I've just told you about. . . . Other programs that assist low-income families with basic needs that compete with the food budget, such as housing, energy, and childcare assistance, are equally vital, particularly in our current economic climate of rising food and energy prices.

The increased SNAP benefit, advocated by many stakeholders, was ultimately supported by the committee and issued to SNAP recipients in April 2009 as part of the American Recovery and Reinvestment Act. Dr Cutts's testimony and Children's HealthWatch data played a small role in making that happen.

The question then arose: did the increase actually make any impact? Children's HealthWatch researchers were recently able to address this question directly in real-time with data collected before, during, and after the SNAP increase. The policy action brief, *Boost to SNAP Benefits Protected Young Children's Health*,[65] (image below) was released in October 2011 and showed that young children in families receiving SNAP after the increase were more likely to be classified as "well" (as defined above) compared to young children in families who were likely eligible but not receiving the benefit. The release was timed to allow consideration by legislators convening for the (now dissolved) Joint Select Committee on Deficit Reduction, charged with reducing the national deficit.

The brief *Boost to SNAP Benefits Protected Young Children's Health* was disseminated to educate all Capitol Hill staff focused on agriculture issues (under which nutrition assistance falls) and policy and legislative contacts nationally and in each Children's HealthWatch city.

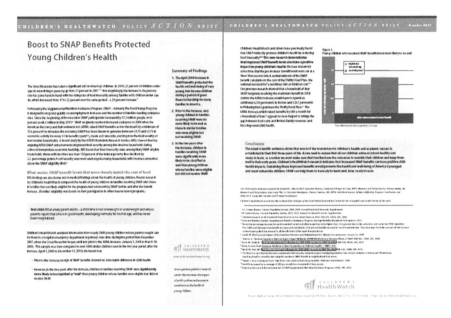

FIGURE 11.2

11.19 LIMITATIONS OF CHILDREN'S HEALTHWATCH FINDINGS

Although the Children's HealthWatch dataset has many strengths, there are certainly limitations. Interviewers are trained to be as professional as possible, properly describe consent procedures, assure the participant of confidentiality, and administer the survey to each participant equally and without bias. However, it is possible that a participant may respond to the survey differently because he or she is in a clinical setting. As with any study, there are also eligible individuals who choose not to participate for their own reasons and other individuals who are not eligible for the study as previously described. Accurate income data other than that based on broad categories of eligibility for public health insurance and other public benefits is difficult to elicit; as a result, the child's insurance status is typically used as a proxy for low-income in Children's HealthWatch analyses (private insurance is used as an exclusion criteria for the analytic dataset).

As with any cross-sectional study design, one cannot determine causal relationships from the findings in any of the studies mentioned. At this time, the Children's HealthWatch sample is not representative of rural populations and no longer collects data from institutions in the western parts of the country. As in many sentinel systems designed for timeliness and early identification of trends, the survey assesses families in emergency departments and hospital-based clinics serving predominantly lower income populations.[66] Therefore, the children represent a group at elevated risk for negative health outcomes and/or developmental risk rather than a random sample of all children in the US. Because the research group is primarily comprised of health professionals rather than economists, the statistical techniques used are derived from public health practice rather than those more commonly used by economists who study hardship and public assistance programs.[5]

11.20   KEY POINTS AND CHILDREN'S HEALTHWATCH RECOMMENDATIONS FOR POLICY ACTION

The body of work by Children's HealthWatch underscores the importance of food security in ensuring healthy growth and development for young children. Funding of SNAP and discretionary programs, like WIC and housing subsidies, targeted to poor families is currently politically contentious. Children's HealthWatch often tries to reframe the discussion by pointing out that the programs should not be viewed as ideological footballs but as effective methods of health promotion; whether or not a family receives assistance from these programs can be the determining factor in a child's overall health and development. While there are other findings not presented here due to space considerations, the research summarized in this paper provides evidence-based support for:

- Maximized and sustained funding for programs like SNAP, WIC, TANF, LIHEAP, and housing subsidy programs.
- Maintenance of program structure for SNAP and other key entitlement programs. Changes to the fundamental structure of these programs would remove their ability to expand in tough economic times and would leave many eligible people without benefits when they need them most.
- Re-evaluation of the use of the Thrifty Food Plan as the basis for SNAP benefit calculations in order to better gauge the true cost of purchasing foods that form a healthy diet; the Low Cost Food Plan is a more realistic reflection of costs in urban communities. This will likely result in an increase in SNAP benefits.

- Reduction or elimination of barriers to key public assistance programs for those who are eligible and want to apply, including legal permanent residents.
- Careful consideration of the impacts of legislation dealing with greenhouse gas emissions and global climate disruption to ensure energy price increases do not fall disproportionately on low-income families.

11.21 DISCUSSION

Children's HealthWatch provides one model of how the clinical and research expertise of pediatric health professionals can be utilized, as the American Academy of Pediatrics urges, to "stand up, speak up, and step up for children."[67] Other leading researchers focus on school-age children, adolescents, and children with special needs and employ a variety of methodologies to assess hardship.[8-11] The pediatric surveillance model is different from those of equally important efforts from other disciplines. Although open to criticism from an econometric perspective, such a model leverages the credibility of pediatricians to gain the attention of policy makers and the public for the youngest, poorest, and most invisible Americans—our young children.

For such children, early deprivation of basic needs may result in poor health and developmental delays that may or may not be remediated later in life. These children struggle in the classroom and, as a result, may incur long-term costs for school and health care systems and later difficulties participating in a competitive global workforce. As we illustrated with the example of Dr Cutts's 2008 testimony before Congress, 2009 increase in SNAP benefit, and our recent 2011 Policy Action Brief linking the increase to positive child health outcomes, good science makes good policy when shared effectively. Scientists can generate credible evidence for other scientists. The challenge is to translate the findings into useful formats for advocates, funders, and policy makers so that accurate information is disseminated, effective policy is proposed, resources are focused, and decision makers understand the impact of their choices based on data rather than ideology. With empirically sound evidence, advocates can bring their concerns to policy makers and educate them about programs that have been shown to decrease America's families' material hardships and suggest budget priorities that might best allocate critical resources to key assistance programs. Working alone, no group will solve children's poverty and multiple hardships. However, working collaboratively each group has a role to play in protecting the health and well-being of young children and their families.

FOOTNOTES

i.   Sentinel samples are subpopulations in which occurrence of a disease indicates or predicts rates in the general population or subpopulations that may be especially vulnerable to a disease and experience higher disease rates before the general population is affected (the "canaries in the coal mine"). They are also subpopulations in which occurrence of or exposure to disease at one age or life-cycle phase may reliably predict disease at later ages or life-cycle phases.

ii. Discretionary programs are funded year to year and are not obligated to serve all those are eligible; TANF, WIC, LIHEAP, and housing subsidies fall into this category.

iii. This question is asked in the National Health Assessment Needs Education Survey III with 5 response alternatives instead of 4. In that version, "very good" is also an option.

iv. We have only included Adjusted Odds Ratios for peer-reviewed publications.

v.   Hospital charges reflect the amount the hospital billed for the entire hospital stay and do not include professional (physician) fees. Costs tend to reflect the actual costs to produce hospital services, while charges represent what the hospital billed for the care.28

vi. Details of the USDA "Thrifty Food Plan" and other food plans are available at www.cnpp.usda.gov/usdafoodplanscostoffood.htm.

REFERENCES

1. Nord M, Andrews M, Carlson S. Household Food Security in the United States, 2008. Washington, DC: Economic Research Service, US Dept of Agriculture; 2009.

2. National Research Council. Food Insecurity and Hunger in the United States: An Assessment of the Measure. Washington, DC: The National Academies Press, 2006.

3. Coleman-Jensen A, Nord M, Andrews M, Carlson S. Household Food Security in the United States in 2010. Washington, DC: Economic Research Service, US Dept of Agriculture; 2011.

4. Frank, DA, Casey PH, Black MM, et al. Cumulative hardship and wellness of low-income, young children: multisite surveillance study. Pediatrics. 2010;125:e1115-e1123.

5. Gundersen C, Kreider B, Pepper J. The economics of food insecurity in the United States. Appl Econ Perspect Policy. 2011;33:281-303.

6. Nord M. Food Insecurity in Households with Children: Prevalence, Severity, and Household Characteristics. Washington, DC: Economic Research Service, US Dept of Agriculture; 2009. EIB-56.

7. Pediatric Nutrition Surveillance System (PedNSS). Centers for Disease Control and Prevention Web site. http://www.cdc.gov/pednss/what_is/pednss/index.htm. Accessed January 18, 2012.

8. Early Childhood Longitudinal Program (ECLS). National Center for Education Statistics Web site. http://nces.ed.gov/ecls/. Accessed January 18, 2012.

9. The Fragile Families and Child Wellbeing Study. Princeton University. Web site. http://www.fragilefamilies.princeton.edu/index.asp. Accessed January 18, 2012.

10. National Health and Nutrition Examination Survey III. Centers for Disease Control and Prevention Web site. http://www.cdc.gov/nchs/nhanes/nh3data.htm. Accessed January 18, 2012.

11. Welfare, children, and families: a three-city study. Johns Hopkins University Web site. http://web.jhu.edu/threecitystudy/index.html. Accessed January 18, 2012.

12. DeNavas-Walt C, Proctor BD, Smith JC, et al. Income, Poverty, and Health Insurance in the United States: 2010. Washington, DC: US Census Bureau; 2011.

13. Cutts D, Ettinger de Cuba S, Coleman S, et al. Childcare settings for low-income children. Poster presented at: Annual Conference of the Pediatric Academic Societies; May 1, 2010; Vancouver, Canada.

14. Wunderlich GS, Norwood JL. Food Insecurity and Hunger in the United States: An Assessment of the Measure. Washington, DC: National Academies Press; 2006.

15. Bickel G, Nord M, Price C, Hamilton W, Cook J. Guide to Measuring Household Food Security, Revised 2000. Alexandria, VA: US Dept of Agriculture, Food and Nutrition Service; 2000.

16. Food security in the United States: definitions of hunger and food security. Economic Research Service Web site. http://www.ers.usda.gov/briefing/foodsecurity/labels.htm. Accessed January 19, 2012.

17. Nord M. ECLS-K 1998-99 food security status file: technical documentation and user notes. Economic Research Service Web site. http://www.ers.usda.gov/Data/foodsecurity/ECLSK/eclsk9899.pdf. Updated February 8, 2001. Accessed January 19, 2012.

18. Cook J, Frank DA, Levenson SM, et al. Child food insecurity increases risks posed by household food insecurity to young children's health. J Nutr. 2006;136:1073-1076.

19. Glascoe FP. Parents' evaluation of developmental status: how well do parents' concerns identify children with behavioral and emotional problems? Clin Pediatr. 2003; 42:133-138.

20. Kemper KJ, Babonis TR. Screening for maternal depression in pediatric clinics. Am J Dis Child. 1992;146:876-878.

21. Cook JT, Frank DA, Berkowitz C, et al. Food insecurity is associated with adverse health outcomes among human infants and toddlers. J Nutr. 2004;134:1432-1438.

22. Casey PH, Szeto K, Lensing S, Bogle M, Weber J. Children in foodinsufficient, low-income families: prevalence, health, and nutrition status. Arch Pediatr Adolesc Med. 2001; 155:508-514.

23. Jyoti DF, Frongillo EA, Jones SJ. Food insecurity affects school children's academic performance, weight gain, and social skills. J Nutr. 2005; 135:2831-2839.

24. Laraia BA, Siega-Riz AM, Gundersen C, Dole N. Psychosocial factors and socioeconomic indicators are associated with household food insecurity among pregnant women. J Nutr. 2006; 136:177-182.

25. Gundersen C, kreider B. Bounding the effects of food insecurity on children's health outcomes. J of Health Econ. 2009; 28:971-983.

26. Healthcare Cost and Utilization Project (HCUP). Agency for Healthcare Research and Quality Web site. http://hcupnet.ahrq.gov/HCUPnet.jsp. Accessed February 13, 2012.

27. Hospitalization in the United States, 2002: HCUP Fact Book No. 6. Agency for Healthcare Research and Quality Web site. http://archive.ahrq.gov/data/hcup/factbk6/ Published June 2005. Accessed February 13, 2012

28. Healthcare Cost and Utilization Project (HCUP). Agency for Healthcare Research and Quality Website. http://www.hcupus.ahrq.gov/reports/factsandfigures/2009/definitions.jsp. Accessed February 13, 2012.

29. Lozoff B, Jimenez E, Hagen J, Mollen E, Wolf AW. Poorer behavioral and developmental outcome more than 10 years after treatment for iron deficiency in infancy. Pediatrics. 2000;105(4):E51.

30. Oppenheimer SJ. Iron and its relation to immunity and infectious disease. J Nutr. 2001;131:616S-633S.

31. Skalicky A, Meyers AF, Adams WG, Yang Z, Cook JT, Frank DA. Child food insecurity and iron deficiency anemia in low-income infants and toddlers in the United States. Matern Child Health J. 2006;10:177-185.

32. Park K, Kersey M, Geppert J, Story M, Cutts D, Himes JH. Household food insecurity is a risk factor for iron-deficiency anaemia in a multi-ethnic, low-income sample of infants and toddlers. Public Health Nutr. 2009;12:2120-2128.

33. Glascoe FP. Collaborating with Parents: Using Parents' Evaluation of Developmental Status to Detect and Address Developmental and Behavioral Problems. Nashville, TN: Ellsworth & Vandermeer Press; 1998.

34. Rose-Jacobs R, Black MM, Casey PH, et al. Household food insecurity: associations with at-risk infant and toddler development. Pediatrics. 2008;121:65-72.

35. Lozoff B, Beard J, Connor J, Barbara F, Georgieff M, Schallert T. Long-lasting neural and behavioral effects of iron deficiency in infancy. Nutr Rev. 2006;64(5 Pt 2):S34-S43.

36. Casey P, Goolsby S, Berkowitz C, et al. Maternal depression, changing public assistance, food security, and child health status. Pediatrics. 2004;113:298-304.

37. Glascoe FP, Leew S. Parenting behaviors, perceptions, and psychosocial risk: impacts on young children's development. Pediatrics. 2010;125:313-319.

38. Yen ST, Andrews M, Chen Z, Eastwood DB. Food Stamp Program participation and food insecurity: an instrumental variables approach. Am J Agr Econ. 2008;90:117-132.

39. Wise, PH. Children of the Recession. Arch Pediatr Adolesc Med. 2009;163:1063-1064.

40. Devaney BL, Ellwood MR, Love JM. Programs that mitigate the effects of poverty on children. Future Child. 1997; 7:88-112.

41. DePolt R, Moffitt RA, Ribar D. Food Stamps, Temporary Assistance for Needy Families and food hardships in three American cities. Pacific Econ Rev. 2009;14:445-473.

42. Chilton M, Black MM, Berkowitz C, et al. Food insecurity and risk of poor health among US-born children of immigrants. Am J Public Health. 2009;99:556-562.

43. Bailey K, Ettinger de Cuba S, Cook JT, March EL, Coleman S, Frank DA. Too many hurdles: barriers to receiving SNAP put children's health at risk. Children's HealthWatch . Published March 2011.

44. Carlson A, Lino M, Juan WY, Hanson K, Basiotis PP. Thrifty Food Plan, 2006. Center for Nutrition Policy and Promotion Web site. http://www.cnpp.usda.gov/Publications/FoodPlans/MiscPubs/TFP2006Re port.pdf. Published April 2007. Accessed December 20, 2011.

45. Thayer J, Murphy C, Cook J, Ettinger de Cuba S, DaCosta R, Chilton M. Coming Up Short: High food costs outstrip food stamp benefits. Children's HealthWatch. Published September 2008.

46. Neault N, Cook JT, Morris V, Frank DA; Boston Medical Center Dept of Pediatrics. The real cost of a healthy diet: healthful foods are out of reach for low-income families in Boston, Massachusetts. Children's HealthWatch. Published August 2005.

47. Breen A, Cahil R, Ettinger de Cuba S, Cook J, Chilton M. The Real Cost of a Healthy Diet. Children's HealthWatch. Published November 2011.

48. WIC program coverage: how many eligible individuals participated in the Special Supplemental Nutrition Program for Women, Infants and Children (WIC): 1994 to 2003? Food and Nutrition Service Web site. http://www.fns.usda.gov/oane/MENU/Published/WIC/FILES/WICEligibles. pdf. Accessed February 8, 2012.

49. WIC At a Glance. Food and Nutrition Service Web site. http://www.fns.usda.gov/wic/aboutwic/wicataglance.htm. Last modified October 12, 2011. Accessed November 8, 2011.

50. Winicki J, Jolliffe D, Gundersen C. How do food assistance programs improve the well-being of low-income families? Washington, DC: Economic Research Service, US Dept of Agriculture; 2002. Food Assistance and Nutrition Research Report No. 26-9.

51. US General Accounting Office. Early intervention: federal investments like WIC can produce savings. Report to Congressional Requesters. GAO/HRD-92-18. April 7, 1992.

52. Jeng K, March EL, Cook JT, Ettinger de Cuba S; Children's HealthWatch. Feeding our future: growing up healthy with WIC. Published March 2009.

53. Cutts DB, Meyers AF, Black MM, et al. US housing insecurity and the health of very young children. Am J Public Health. 2011;101:1508-1514.

54. Meyers A, Cutts D, Frank D et al. Subsidized housing and children's nutritional status: data from a multisite surveillance study. Arch Pediatr Adolsc Med. 2005;159;551-556.

55. March EL, Ettinger de Cuba S, Gayman A, et al; Children's Health Watch; Medical-Legal Partnership/Boston. RX for hunger: affordable housing. Children's HealthWatch Report. Published December 2009.

56. Frank DA, Roos N, Meyers A, et al. Seasonal variation in weight-forage in a pediatric emergency room. Public Health Rep. 1996;111:366-371.

57. Cook JT, Frank DA, Casey PH, et al. A brief indicator of household energy security: associations with food security, child health, and child development in US infants and toddlers. Pediatrics. 2008;122:e867-e875.

58. Frank DA, Neault NB, Skalicky A, et al. Heat or eat: the Low Income Home Energy Assistance Program and nutritional and health risks among children less than 3 years of age. Pediatrics. 2006;118:e1293-e1302.

59. Bailey K, Ettinger de Cuba S, Cook JT, March EL Coleman S, Frank DA. LIHEAP Stabilizes family housing and protects children's health. Children's HealthWatch Policy Action Brief. Published February 2011.

60. Agénor M, Ettinger de Cuba S, Rose-Jacobs R, Frank DA. Impact of food insecurity on the development of young low-income Black and Latino children. Children's HealthWatch & The Joint Center for Political and Economic Studies Health Policy Institute. May 2006.

61. Gayman A, Ettinger de Cuba S, Cook JT, et al. Earning more, receiving less: loss of benefits and child hunger. Children's HealthWatch Report. Published September 2010.

62. March E, Cook JT, Ettinger de Cuba S, Gayman A, Frank DA. Healthy families in hard times: solutions for multiple family hardships. Children's HealthWatch. http://www.childrenshealthwatch.org/upload/resource/multiplehardships_re port_jun10.pdf?PHPSESSID=09d6af013d992dfbaac29b48c97a6e8b. Published June 2010.

63. US House Committee on Agriculture. Subcommittee reviews the cost of hunger in America. http://agriculture.house.gov/press/PRArticle.aspx?NewsID=384. July 23, 2008. Accessed September, 15 2011.

64. US House Committee on Agriculture. Hearing to review short and long term costs of hunger in America. http://agriculture.house.gov/testimony/110/110-43.pdf. July 23, 2008. Accessed September 15, 2011.

65. March EL, Ettinger de Cuba S, Bailey K, et al. Boost to SNAP benefits protected young children's health. Children's HealthWatch Web. Published October 2011.

66. Substance Abuse and Mental Health Services Administration. Drug Abuse Warning Network, 2009: Methodology Report. Rockville, MD: Substance Abuse and Mental Health Services Administration, US Dept of Health and Human Services; 2011.

67. AAP leader says to stand up, speak up, and step up for child health [news release]. Boston, MA: American Academy of Pediatrics; October 11, 2008. http://www2.aap.org/press-room/nce/nce08childhealth.htm. Accessed January 1, 2012.

Keywords

- Food security
- Food insecurity
- Malnutrition
- Under-nutrition
- Hunger
- Starvation
- Obesity
- Measurement
- Child malnutrition
- Stunting
- Household food insecurity
- Africa
- Adolescent
- Child
- Epidemiology
- Food
- Hunger
- Social determinants of health
- Food insecurity
- Aboriginal peoples
- First nations Mйtis
- Child obesity
- Canada
- Income
- Food (in)security
- Urban poor
- Child health
- Stunting

- **Malnutrition**
- **Wealth status**
- **Nairobi**
- **Kenya**

Author Notes

Chapter 3

Acknowledgements
We acknowledge the valuable contributions of staff of the NUHDSS and the Maternal Child Health/Indepth Vaccination Projects at the African Population and Health Research Center (APHRC). We particularly acknowledge Martin Mutua who supported the data management. Moreover, we acknowledge the two reviewers, Anu Rammohan and Chrissie Thakwalakwa for their thoughtful comments and suggestions that greatly improved the manuscript. This research was supported by the Consortium for Advanced Research Training in Africa (CARTA). CARTA is jointly led by the African Population and Health Research Center and the University of the Witwatersrand and is funded by the Wellcome Trust (UK) (Grant No: 087547/Z/08/Z); the Department for International Development (DfID) under the Development Partnerships in Higher Education (DelPHE); the Carnegie Corporation of New York (Grant No: B 8606); the Ford Foundation (Grant No: 1100–0399); Google.Org (Grant No: 191994); Sida (Grant No: 54100029); and MacArthur Foundation Grant No: 10-95915-000-INP. The Urbanization, Poverty, and Health Dynamics (UPHD) research project was funded by the Wellcome Trust (Grant Number GR 07830 M). The Monitoring and assessing the impact of immunization and other childhood interventions, an INDEPTH Network collaboration project was funded by the Danish Development Agency (DANIDA) (DFC Project no 09-09-105SSI). This research was also made possible through the generous funding for the NUHDSS by a number of donors including the Rockefeller Foundation (USA), the Wellcome Trust (UK), the William and Flora Hewlett Foundation (USA), Comic Relief (UK), the Swedish International Development Cooperation (SIDA) and the Bill and Melinda Gates Foundation (USA) and the core funding for APHRC by the William and Flora Hewlett Foundation (Grant# 2009–40510), and the Swedish International Cooperation Agency (SIDA) (Grant# 2011–001578).

Competing Interests
The authors declare no conflicts of interest.

Authors' Contributions

MM conducted the literature review, analysis and interpretation of data as well as drafted the initial manuscript; NK contributed to the conceptualisation of the study and reviewed the manuscript for substantial intellectual content. He also guided the methods and analysis; MN contributed to the conceptualisation of the study and reviewed the manuscript for substantial intellectual content. He also provided close supervision throughout the process; CK contributed to the conceptualisation of the study and reviewed the manuscript for substantial intellectual content. She provided guidance on the analysis and the discussion. All authors have read and approved the final manuscript.

Chapter 4

Acknowledgements

MAL-ED Network Investigators by region: Africa: In South Africa: Pascal Bessong (University of Venda, Thohoyandou, South Africa), Angelina Mapula (University of Venda, Thohoyandou, South Africa), Emanuel Nyathi (University of Venda, Thohoyandou, South Africa), Cloupas Mahopo (University of Venda, Thohoyandou, South Africa), Amidou Samie (University of Venda, Thohoyandou, South Africa), Cebisa Nesamvuni (University of Venda, Thohoyandou, South Africa); In Tanzania: Erling Svensen (Haydom Lutheran Hospital, University of Bergen, Norway), Estomih R. Mduma (Haydom Lutheran Hospital, Haydom, Tanzania), Crystal L. Patil (University of Illinois, Urbana-Champaign, IL, USA), Caroline Amour (Haydom Lutheran Hospital, Haydom, Tanzania): South America: In Brazil: Aldo A. M. Lima (Universidade Federal do Ceara, Fortaleza, Brazil), Reinaldo B. Oriá (Universidade Federal do Ceara, Fortaleza, Brazil), Noélia L. Lima (Universidade Federal do Ceara, Fortaleza, Brazil), Alberto M. Soares, (Universidade Federal do Ceara, Fortaleza, Brazil), Alexandre H. Bindá (Universidade Federal do Ceara, Fortaleza, Brazil), Ila F. N. Lima (Universidade Federal do Ceara, Fortaleza, Brazil), Josiane S. Quetz (Universidade Federal do Ceara, Fortaleza, Brazil), Milena L. Moraes (Universidade Federal do Ceara, Fortaleza, Brazil). Bruna L. L. Maciel (Universidade Federal do Ceara, Fortaleza, Brazil), Hilda Costa (Universidade Federal do Ceara, Fortaleza, Brazil), Jose Quirino Filho (Universidade Federal do Ceara, Fortaleza, Brazil), Álvaro J. M. Leite (Universidade Federal do Ceara, Fortaleza, Brazil), Francisco B. Mota (Universidade Federal do Ceara, Fortaleza, Brazil), Alessandra F. Di Moura (Universidade Federal do Ceara, Fortaleza, Brazil); In Peru: Maribel Paredes Olortegui (A.B. PRISMA, Iquitos, Peru), Cesar Banda Chavez (A.B. PRISMA, Iquitos, Peru), Dixner Rengifo Trigoso

(A.B. PRISMA, Iquitos, Peru), Julian Torres Flores (A.B. PRISMA, Iquitos, Peru), Angel Orbe Vasquez (A.B. PRISMA, Iquitos, Peru), Silvia Rengifo Pinedo (A.B. PRISMA, Iquitos, Peru), Angel Mendez Acosta (A.B. PRISMA, Iquitos, Peru); South Asia: In Bangladesh: Tahmeed Ahmed (ICDDR-B, Dhaka, Bangladesh), Rashidul Haque (ICDDR-B, Dhaka, Bangladesh), AM Shamsir Ahmed (ICDDR-B, Dhaka, Bangladesh), Munirul Islam, (ICDDR-B, Dhaka, Bangladesh), Iqbal Hossain (ICDDR-B, Dhaka, Bangladesh), Mustafa Mahfuz (ICDDR-B, Dhaka, Bangladesh), Dinesh Mondol (ICDDR-B, Dhaka, Bangladesh), Fahmida Tofail (ICDDR-B, Dhaka, Bangladesh); In India: Gagandeep Kang (Christian Medical College, Vellore, India), Sushil John (Christian Medical College, Vellore, India), Sudhir Babji (Christian Medical College, Vellore, India), Mohan Venkata Raghava (Christian Medical College, Vellore, India), Anuradha Rose (Christian Medical College, Vellore, India), Beena Kurien (Christian Medical College, Vellore, India), Anuradha Bose (Christian Medical College, Vellore, India), Jayaprakash Muliyil (Christian Medical College, Vellore, India), Anup Ramachandran (Christian Medical College, Vellore, India); In Nepal: Carl J Mason (Armed Forces Research Institute of Medical Sciences, Bangkok, Thailand), Prakash Sunder Shrestha (Institute of Medicine, Tribuhvan University, Kathmandu, Nepal), Sanjaya Kumar Shrestha (Walter Reed/AFRIMS Research Unit, Kathmandu, Nepal), Ladaporn Bodhidatta, (Armed Forces Research Institute of Medical Sciences, Bangkok, Thailand), Ram Krishna Chandyo (Institute of Medicine, Tribuhvan University, Kathmandu, Nepal), Rita Shrestha (Institute of Medicine, Tribuhvan University, Kathmandu, Nepal), Binob Shrestha (Walter Reed/AFRIMS Research Unit, Kathmandu), Tor Strand (University of Bergen, Bergen, Norway), Manjeswori Ulak (Institute of Medicine, Tribuhvan University, Kathmandu, Nepal); In Pakistan: Zulfiqar A Bhutta (Aga Khan University, Naushahro Feroze, Pakistan), Anita K M Zaidi (Aga Khan University, Naushahro Feroze, Pakistan), Sajid Soofi (Aga Khan University, Naushahro Feroze, Pakistan), Ali Turab (Aga Khan University, Naushahro Feroze, Pakistan), Didar Alam (Aga Khan University, Naushahro Feroze, Pakistan), Shahida Qureshi (Aga Khan University, Naushahro Feroze, Pakistan), Aisha K Yousafzai (Aga Khan University, Naushahro Feroze, Pakistan), Asad Ali (Aga Khan University, Naushahro Feroze, Pakistan), Imran Ahmed (Aga Khan University, Naushahro Feroze, Pakistan), Sajad Memon (Aga Khan University, Naushahro Feroze, Pakistan), Muneera Rasheed (Aga Khan University, Naushahro Feroze, Pakistan); North America: In the United States: Michael Gottlieb (Foundation for the NIH, Bethesda, MD, USA), Mark Miller (Fogarty International Center/National Institutes of Health, Bethesda,

MD, USA), Karen H. Tountas (Foundation for the NIH, Bethesda, MD, USA), Rebecca Blank (Foundation for the NIH, Bethesda, MD, USA), Dennis Lang, (Fogarty International Center/National Institutes of Health, Bethesda, MD, USA), Stacey Knobler (Fogarty International Center/National Institutes of Health, Bethesda, MD, USA), Monica McGrath (Fogarty International Center/National Institutes of Health, Bethesda, MD, USA), Stephanie Richard (Fogarty International Center/National Institutes of Health, Bethesda, MD, USA), Jessica Seidman (Fogarty International Center/National Institutes of Health, Bethesda, MD, USA), Zeba Rasmussen (Fogarty International Center/National Institutes of Health, Bethesda, MD, USA), Ramya Ambikapathi (Fogarty International Center/National Institutes of Health, Bethesda, MD, USA), Benjamin McCormick (Fogarty International Center/National Institutes of Health, Bethesda, MD, USA), Stephanie Psaki (Fogarty International Center/National Institutes of Health, Bethesda, MD, USA), Vivek Charu (Fogarty International Center/National Institutes of Health, Bethesda, MD, USA), Jhanelle Graham (Fogarty International Center/National Institutes of Health, Bethesda, MD, USA), Gaurvika Nayyar (Fogarty International Center/National Institutes of Health, Bethesda, MD, USA), Viyada Doan (Fogarty International Center/National Institutes of Health, Bethesda, MD, USA), Leyfou Dabo (Fogarty International Center/National Institutes of Health, Bethesda, MD, USA), Danny Carreon (Fogarty International Center/National Institutes of Health, Bethesda, MD, USA), Archana Mohale (Fogarty International Center/National Institutes of Health, Bethesda, MD, USA), Christel Host (Fogarty International Center/National Institutes of Health, Bethesda, MD, USA), Dick Guerrant (University of Virginia, Charlottesville, VA, USA), Bill Petri (University of Virginia, Charlottesville, VA, USA), Eric Houpt (University of Virginia, Charlottesville, VA, USA), Jean Gratz (University of Virginia, Charlottesville, VA, USA), Leah Barrett (University of Virginia, Charlottesville, VA, USA), Rebecca Scharf (University of Virginia, Charlottesville, VA, USA), Laura Caulfield (Johns Hopkins University, Baltimore, MD, USA), William Checkley (Johns Hopkins University, Baltimore, MD, USA), Margaret Kosek (Johns Hopkins University, Baltimore, MD, USA), Pablo Penataro Yori (Johns Hopkins University, Baltimore, MD, USA), Gwenyth Lee (Johns Hopkins University, Baltimore, MD, USA), Ping Chen (Johns Hopkins University, Baltimore, MD, USA), Robert Black (Johns Hopkins University, Baltimore, MD, USA), Laura Murray-Kolb (Pennsylvania State University, University Park, PA, USA), Barbara Schaefer (Pennsylvania State University, University Park, PA, USA), William Pan (Duke University, Durham, NC, USA).

Funding

The Etiology, Risk Factors and Interactions of Enteric Infections and Malnutrition and the Consequences for Child Health and Development Project (MAL-ED) is carried out as a collaborative project supported by the Bill & Melinda Gates Foundation. William Checkley was further supported by a Clinician Scientist Award from the Johns Hopkins University and a K99/R00 Pathway to Independence Award (K99HL096955) from the National Heart, Lung and Blood Institute, National Institutes of Health.

Competing Interests

The authors declare that they have no competing interests.

Authors' Contributions

SP and WC contributed equally to the conception, design and analysis of data, interpretation of findings, and writing of manuscript. ZB participated in study conception, design and data acquisition, and a critical review of the manuscript. JS, SR, MMc, LC, MMi participated in study design and critical review of the manuscript. TA, SA, PB, MI, SJ, MK, AL, CN, PS, and ES contributed to study design and data acquisition. WC had ultimate oversight over the study design, data analysis and writing of this manuscript. All authors read and approved the final manuscript.

Chapter 5

Acknowledgements

The Jimma Longitudinal Family Survey of Youth was funded by the Packard Foundation, Campton Foundation, National Institute of Health and National Science Foundation. We are extremely grateful to adolescents involved in the study, data collectors and the research team members, Prof.Dennis Hogan, Dr. Kifle Woldemichael, Prof. Challi Jira and Mr. Fasil Tesema.

Competing Interests

The authors declare that they have no competing interests.

Authors' Contributions

The authors' responsibilities were as follows: DL, CH, TB & AG: Designed and supervised the study and ensured quality of the data and made a substantial contribution to the local implementation of the study and PK, CH, WK & DL assisted in the analysis and interpretation of the data. All authors critically reviewed the manuscript. TB, the corresponding author did the analysis & drafted the manuscript and had the responsibility to submit the manuscript for publication. All authors read and approved the final manuscript.

Chapter 6

Acknowledgments
The authors thank all our participants from the community of Kwale District in the Coast Province of Kenya. This work was supported, in part, by Grants-in-Aid for Scientific Research (KAKENHI) (A) 252575030001 and (B) 22406023 from the Ministry of Education, Culture, Sports, Science and Technology of Japan (MEXT) and by the Graduate School of International Health Development, Nagasaki University. This paper is published with the permission of the Director of KEMRI.

Competing Interests
The authors declare that they have no competing interests.

Authors' Contributions
CS and SK: responsible for the overall research plan, the coordination of the nutrition survey, data analyses, and writing the manuscript; MM: provided technical support for the study design and data analyses; MK: provided technical support and coordinated the nutrition survey; JT: provided technical support for the implementation of the nutrition survey and data analyses; MC: provided technical support for the implementation of the survey in the community. All authors read and approved the final manuscript.

Chapter 7

Acknowledgments
We acknowledge members of the HBSC study in Canada and cross-nationally. International coordinator of the HBSC study is Dr. Candace Currie, University of St. Andrews, Scotland. The international databank manager is Dr. Oddrun Samdal, University of Bergen, Norway. The Canadian principal investigators of HBSC are Drs. John Freeman and William Pickett, Queen's University, and its national coordinator is Matthew King. We thank Nathan King and Jessica Byrnes for their work in formatting this manuscript for submission. This analysis was supported by an operating grant from the Canadian Institutes of Health Research (MOP 130379, principal investigator CD).

Chapter 8

Funding

This study was supported by grants from Quebec's Ministry of Health and Social Services, the Quebec Fund for Research on Society and Culture (Fonds québécois de la recherche sur la société et la culture), the Quebec Fund for Research on Nature and Technology (Fonds québécois de la recherche sur la nature et la technologie), the Health Research Fund of Quebec (Fonds de recherche en santé du Québec), Quebec's Ministry of Research, Science, and Technology, the Canadian Institutes of Health Research, the Social Sciences and Humanities Research Council of Canada, Human Resources Development Canada, Health Canada, the Lucie and André Chagnon Foundation, the National Science Foundation, the University of Montreal, Laval University, and McGill University. The funders supported the design and conduct of the study; collection, management, and analysis of the data, but had no influence on the preparation, review, or approval of the manuscript. MM is the recipient of a Young Researcher Award from the French National Research Agency. MB is supported by the Canada Research Chair program. The funders had no role in data analysis, decision to publish, or preparation of the manuscript.

Competing Interests

The authors have declared that no competing interests exist.

Acknowledgments

We are grateful to the parents and children of the Québec Longitudinal Study of Child Development (QLSCD). We thank the Québec Institute of Statistics, Mireille Jetté, and the GRIP staff for data collection and management.

Author Contributions

Conceived and designed the experiments: MM JFC SC RT MB. Analyzed the data: MM JFC. Contributed reagents/materials/analysis tools: MM JFC BF CG SC RT MB. Wrote the paper: MM JFC BF CG SC RT MB

Chapter 9

Acknowledgements

The Québec portion of this study has been partly financed by the Canadian Institute of Health Research. The analyses were performed using data from the Québec Longitudinal Study of Child Development (1998-2010) (QLSCD), conducted by Santé Québec, a division of the Institut de la Statistique du Québec (ISQ) and funded by the Ministry of Health and Social Services of Québec. In Jamaica, the analyses were performed using data from the Jamaica Youth Risk and Resiliency Behaviour Survey 2005, conducted by the Sir Arthur Lewis Institute of Social and Economic Studies with funding from the USAID and Ministry of Health Jamaica. Technical assistance was provided by MEASURE Evaluation, Tulane University.

Competing Interests

The authors declare that they have no competing interests.

Authors' Contributions

LD is the principal investigator and was primarily responsible for the conceptualization of the study. DF, DB, and MG analyzed the data, and DF, DB, and FT wrote the manuscript. GGS, KF, and RW critically revised the manuscript for important intellectual content. All authors read and approved the final manuscript.

Chapter 10

Acknowledgments

The authors would like acknowledge the assistance of Lin Yuan of the Southwest Ontario Aboriginal Health Access Centre, Allison and Michelle Gates, and Earnest Matton (Little Brown Bear). Funding for this research was provided by the Canadian Institutes of Health Research.

Competing Interests

The authors declare that they have no competing interests.

Authors' Contributions

JB contributed the focus of the paper, conducted the literature review and data analysis and wrote the first draft. MC assisted with the qualitative data collection and commented and revised the paper and is PI on the supporting grant. RH contributed to the conceptualization of the paper, revised the method for data analysis and commented on later drafts. PW supervised the qualitative data collection and is co-PI on the supporting grant, and SG collaborated on the data collection design and facilitated community access. All authors read and approved the final manuscript.

Chapter 11

Acknowledgements

We are grateful to the families who participated in this study, and the staff in emergency departments and primary care centers that have permitted us to work with their patients. We thank current and past principal investigators Maureen Black, PhD; Timothy Heeren, MD; Diana Cutts, MD; Patrick Casey, MD; Alan Meyers, MD, MPH; Nieves Zaldivar, MD; Martha Wellman, MD; and Carol Berkowitz, MD; for their dedication to this project. We also thank all of the dedicated Children's HealthWatch interviewers, site coordinators, data analysts, and financial administrators past and present; Ingrid Weiss, MS; Chenelle Christian and Tu Quan, MPH, for bibliographic assistance; Elizabeth March, MCP, as Executive Director emeritus; and Zhaoyan Yang, MA, and Sharon Coleman, MS, for their data management and analysis support. Children's HealthWatch's work on behalf of underserved young children would not be possible without the generous support of private foundations and individual donors. Past and current donors include: Annie E. Casey Foundation, Anthony Spinazzola Foundation, Candle Foundation, Citizens Energy Corporation, Claneil Foundation, Daniel Pitino Foundation, Eos Foundation, Feeding America (formerly America's Second Harvest), Fireman Foundation, Gold Foundation, Gryphon Fund, Beatrice Fox Auerbach Foundation Fund at the Hartford Foundation for Public Giving, Joint Center for Political and Economic Studies Health Policy Institute, The Krupp Family Foundation, Larson Family Foundation, Leaves of Grass Fund, The John D. and Catherine T. MacArthur Foundation, MAZON: A Jewish Response to Hunger, National Fuel Funds Network, New Hampshire Charitable Foundation, Pew Charitable Trusts, Project Bread—The Walk For Hunger, Sandpiper Philanthropic Foundation, Thomas Wilson Sanitarium for Children of Baltimore City, United States Department of Agriculture, Vitamin Litigation Funding, private donors and major funding from the W.K. Kellogg Foundation.

Index

T - #0835 - 101024 - C292 - 229/152/13 - PB - 9781774636879 - Gloss Lamination